T0356755

AFTER
DOBBS

AFTER

HOW THE SUPREME COURT

DOBBS

ENDED *ROE* BUT NOT ABORTION

DAVID S. COHEN AND CAROLE JOFFE

BEACON PRESS, BOSTON

BEACON PRESS
Boston, Massachusetts
www.beacon.org

Beacon Press books
are published under the auspices of
the Unitarian Universalist Association of Congregations.

28 27 26 25   8 7 6 5 4 3 2 1

This book is printed on acid-free paper that meets the uncoated paper
ANSI/NISO specifications for permanence as revised in 1992.

Text design and composition by Kim Arney

Library of Congress Cataloging-in-Publication Data
is available for this title.
ISBN: 978-0-8070-1766-1; e-book: 978-0-8070-1765-4;
audiobook: 978-0-8070-1863-7

To those fighting
for reproductive freedom

CONTENTS

AFTER
DOBBS

INTRODUCTION

OHIO

Sometime in May 2022, a ten-year-old girl was raped in Ohio. And then, sometime after that, the girl found out she was pregnant.[1]

Given her age, the circumstances, and her wishes, she and her family decided she would have an abortion. Had they made the decision just days earlier, they would have encountered hurdles for getting an abortion in Ohio, but they could have been overcome. For instance, Ohio had required minors to obtain the written consent of a parent before getting an abortion, but this requirement wouldn't have posed a problem for the minor. Her parent supported her care, so she would have been able to obtain the consent and then care at one of the clinics or hospitals in Ohio that performed abortions. She would have done so, presumably, without the rest of the world finding out about her story. However, because she sought her abortion on June 29, 2022, rather than a week earlier, events took an entirely different turn.

Instead, this girl's story became one of the first known tragedies of the Supreme Court's decision to overrule *Roe v. Wade*. On June 24, just days before the ten-year-old sought an abortion, the Court decided *Dobbs v. Jackson Women's Health Organization*.[2] And that changed everything.

On that Friday morning, the Court announced its decision the same way it had been announcing all of its decisions in the Covid era—by releasing them not in person but rather on the Court website. With several opinions still left to be released for the term and the blockbuster Second Amendment case *New York State Rifle and Pistol Association v. Bruen*[3] having been released the day before, there were many people, including both of us, who thought the Supreme Court was going to wait to release *Dobbs* until the next week, possibly even the last day of its term. Issuing too many ground-shifting decisions that tracked the conservative agenda in rapid succession might not be the look the Court wanted.

We were all wrong. After issuing a decision at 10:01 a.m. eastern time about Medicare reimbursement that featured two of the Court's conservatives joining the Court's three liberals, as had become its custom, the Court let ten minutes pass before posting its next decision on its website. At 10:11 a.m. *Dobbs* appeared on the Court's list of decided cases, and the moment antiabortion activists had been waiting nearly half a century for had arrived. Clicking on the link revealed what we had all suspected—the Court, voting on ideological lines, had overturned *Roe v. Wade*.

For the ten-year-old girl's purposes, this decision on Friday morning could not have come at a worse time and she could not have lived in a worse state. Whereas many other states took days or even weeks to sort out the consequences of the decision, Ohio took less than an hour. Just forty-five minutes after the Supreme Court released its opinion, Ohio attorney general Dave Yost filed a motion in Ohio federal court asking it to allow Ohio to enforce its ban on abortions after six weeks of pregnancy. That ban, passed in 2019, had been put on hold by an Ohio federal judge because it violated the right to abortion from *Roe* and its follow-up case, *Planned Parenthood of Southeastern Pennsylvania v. Casey*.[4] In his motion filed that morning, Yost asked the court to immediately overturn its previous decision that had put the 2019 ban on hold. "The ruling in *Dobbs*," Yost wrote, "represents a substantial change in the law."

Later that day, the court agreed with Yost. Ruling just after 6 p.m. that evening, the federal judge lifted the injunction that had stopped the 2019 law from taking effect. Reflecting the gravity of the moment, the judge wrote that the Supreme Court's overruling of *Roe* meant the judge needed to take "immediate action."[5] As a result of this decision, by Friday evening, barely eight hours after *Dobbs* was released, Ohio became the first state in the country to have an abortion ban restored. Five days later, several Ohio abortion clinics asked the state supreme court to stop the ban, but the court did not act on that request.

This legal wrangling taking place in Ohio's state and federal courts probably went unnoticed by the ten-year-old and her family. However, these decisions had an almost immediate impact on their lives. The abortion ban now in place had no exception for rape and prohibited abortions after the detection of what the law called a "fetal heartbeat," even though there is nothing medical professionals would ordinarily call a heartbeat early in pregnancy. It explained further that an abortion provider must determine if there is "cardiac activity," which occurs at around six weeks of pregnancy.

But six weeks of pregnancy is not what most people typically think it is. Pregnancy is dated from the start of the last menstrual period, so a pregnancy that is six weeks along is often, if the person has a regular menstrual cycle, only four weeks after conception and two weeks after missing a period. In other words, with the Ohio law now in place, people* in the state had a very short time to navigate the obstacle course of finding out they were pregnant: making a decision to get an abortion, finding a clinic, getting an appointment, complying with all of the state requirements for an abortion, and then having the abortion.[6]

For this ten-year-old girl, it was now too late. She went to see a doctor in Ohio on the Monday following the Supreme Court decision. But because *Dobbs* had been decided three days prior to that visit rather than, say, three days after it, the doctor couldn't help her get an abortion in her home state: according to media reports, she was just a few days past her state's now-in-effect six-week limit.

So the ten-year old, with parental help, did what many people had to do after *Dobbs*: she traveled to another state where abortion remained legal. For this girl, that meant going to Indiana. There, she had her abortion and was able to move on to dealing with the trauma of being raped, but without also dealing with being pregnant and eventually giving birth at such a young age.

Ordinarily, that would have been the end of the story about her abortion, and nothing about it would have been publicly known. However, on July 1, one week after *Dobbs* was decided, the *Indianapolis Star* published an article about abortion patients traveling to Indiana for abortion care now that states near Indiana, like Ohio, had criminalized abortion.[7] The article started with a brief anecdote told by Dr. Caitlin Bernard, an

---

*Throughout this book we use both "woman" and "person" to describe who receives an abortion, recognizing the reality that some people who do not identify as women receive abortions, including transgender men and gender-nonconforming individuals. We believe this accomplishes the twin goals of being inclusive but also reflecting the reality that cisgender women receive most abortions. See Loretta J. Ross and Rickie Solinger, *Reproductive Justice: An Introduction* (Oakland: University of California Press, 2017), 6–8; see also Rachel K. Jones and Elizabeth Witwer, "Transgender Abortion Patients and the Provision of Transgender-Specific Care at Non-Hospital Facilities That Provide Abortions," Guttmacher Institute, Jan. 2020.

obstetrician-gynecologist who practices in Indianapolis. Dr. Bernard relayed the story of taking the call from the ten-year-old's Ohio doctor and then the girl coming to Indianapolis, where Dr. Bernard performed her abortion. There were no other details.

Nonetheless, the story went viral. Scores of news outlets around the United States and the world ran with it, no doubt partly because it is a tragically sad story but also because it drove home the harm of *Dobbs* with about as sympathetic a victim as possible. President Joe Biden even weighed in while talking about the Supreme Court and the future of abortion. He said, with increasing emphasis and passion as he spoke, "Just last week it was reported that a ten-year-old girl was a rape victim in Ohio. Ten years old! And she was forced to . . . travel out of the state to Indiana to seek to terminate the pregnancy and maybe save her life—that last part is my judgment, ten years old. Ten years old!—raped, six weeks pregnant, already traumatized, was forced to travel to another state. Imagine being that little girl. Just, I'm serious, just imagine being that little girl. Ten years old!"

Because of this story's power, it immediately drew backlash. Antiabortion politicians and news outlets asked whether the story was true or merely made up out of whole cloth by someone they accused of being merely an abortion rights activist. They insisted that if these events had actually taken place, certainly a parent or a doctor would have reported the horrific crime and there would be a record of an arrest or an investigation. These critics looked foolish later in July when Ohio authorities arrested the alleged rapist and confirmed that the girl had an abortion on June 30, the day before the initial report was published. In July 2023, after pleading guilty, the man was sentenced to life in prison.

Other attacks from the antiabortion movement were lobbed at the doctor who initially spoke to the press about the case. She was accused of violating the patient's privacy and failing to report the rape. Todd Rokita, the vehemently antiabortion Indiana attorney general, spoke out publicly against her, calling for her to be investigated. However, her employer released a statement that she had complied with patient privacy laws, and state health officials released a document showing that she had properly reported the abortion and the abuse.

That didn't stop the harassment, though. Nor the legal action. In November, Rokita filed a complaint with the state medical licensing board against Dr. Bernard alleging that she had violated state privacy law and failed to immediately report child abuse. Dr. Bernard disputed both claims, but in June 2023, the board found that, although she had properly reported the child abuse, she had not followed state privacy law. As a result, the board reprimanded her and fined her $3,000. Later in 2023, the Indiana Supreme Court publicly reprimanded Rokita for his statements about Dr. Bernard.[8]

ARIZONA

Ellie was married with a one-year-old when she found out that she was pregnant again.[9] She had been using an IUD to avoid getting pregnant, but her husband didn't want her using any form of birth control. This was part of a larger pattern of abuse by her husband that included physical abuse and almost strangling Ellie to death at one point. Ellie had secretly obtained an IUD, but when her husband realized she had it, he was furious. Concerned about his anger turning into abuse, she had it removed.

Without birth control, Ellie got pregnant. After feeling unusually nauseated, Ellie snuck to the store to get a pregnancy test, and the result was positive. When she told her husband that she was pregnant but didn't want to have another child, he demanded she not have an abortion. The physical abuse increased.

Nonetheless, Ellie knew she had to have an abortion. Because of the abuse, her marriage was not, in her words, "salvageable." But she knew that if she had another child with her husband, it would be harder for her to leave. "I feel like I'd still be trapped," she said. The best evidence we have about this phenomenon supports Ellie's intuition: women who are not able to access a wanted abortion are more likely to be tethered to their abusive partners.[10] Ellie didn't want this to happen to her, so she needed to find a place to get an abortion.

Ellie lived in Arizona, where prior to *Dobbs* there were eight abortion clinics. After *Dobbs*, though, there was immediate confusion over whether abortion was legal. An 1864 law, updated and codified in 1901, from before Arizona was a state, criminalized abortion, but that had been put on hold while *Roe v. Wade* was good law. Once *Roe* was overruled, all but one of the Arizona clinics decided to close or suspend services out of fear that the state would enforce the old law. A few clinics began offering abortion later in the summer, when a federal judge put a different Arizona law on hold that granted "personhood" status to fetuses. However, not all clinics did this, and at the end of the summer, a state court ruled that this old law could take effect, banning abortion in the entire state. That ruling was overturned in October, when an appeals court ruled that a more recently passed ban on abortion at fifteen weeks superseded the old law, meaning abortion would now be legal in Arizona up to fifteen weeks.[11]

Ellie was looking to have an abortion at the precise time when the clinics were closed in Arizona. With the back-and-forth over the legal status of abortion in her home state and clinics suspending services—some of them reopening and then all being forced to stop abortion until October—the safest route for Ellie to get an abortion, both legally and for her own physical safety, was to leave the state. If she stayed in Arizona, Ellie was considering how she could have an abortion on her own, but she worried that she would hurt herself. Ellie's husband controlled their finances, so she had no access to money of her own. She was able to get financial help from her sympathetic brother-in-law and bought one-way plane tickets for herself and her son to go to Colorado, where her parents live. Ellie has been in Colorado ever since.

Once there, Ellie was able to get an appointment with a doctor who helped her. The doctor worked with his colleague to find funding for Ellie's abortion, and she had a medication abortion at seven weeks along in her pregnancy. Ellie said it was "something I had to do." And in Colorado it remained legal for her to do so, even post-*Dobbs*.

TEXAS

In the spring of 2022, Amanda Zurawski and her husband celebrated that Amanda was finally pregnant.[12] The couple, who had known each other since preschool and had been married for three years, had been through eighteen months of fertility treatments after Amanda learned that she was not ovulating. After exploratory procedures, many medications, and intrauterine insemination, the two were, according to Amanda, "beyond thrilled" that the "grueling" fertility treatment had worked.

In August 2022, barely two months after *Roe* was overturned and about four months into the pregnancy, everything had been going fine. They found out they were having a girl and named her Willow. Amanda was just finishing some preparation for the baby shower her sister was going to throw for her when she began experiencing strange symptoms. She told her doctor, who asked her to come in immediately. A quick examination revealed terrible news—Amanda had an "incompetent cervix" that had dilated early, at seventeen weeks and six days of pregnancy. There was no way she was going to be able to stay pregnant long enough to reach fetal viability, the point at which a fetus could likely survive outside the womb, so the doctors told Amanda that her baby was not going to survive.

If abortion had still been legal before viability, as it was under *Roe v. Wade*, Amanda would have had an abortion. However, because Texas now had a ban on abortion at all stages of pregnancy, she couldn't get the care she sought. Amanda's doctors told her she wasn't yet sick enough to qualify under the state's exception for when a pregnancy threatens the life of the person who is pregnant. She was sent home to wait, knowing that she was being forced to continue a nonviable pregnancy. That night Amanda's water broke, so she returned to the hospital, where she was diagnosed with preterm premature rupture of the membranes. The proper treatment was, once again, for her to have an abortion, but because Willow still had a heartbeat and Amanda was not experiencing any major illness, there was still nothing her doctors could do for her.

Amanda considered traveling to another state, but she realized that was impossible, given her situation. She lived in the middle of Texas, so it would be more than an eight-hour drive to get to a state where abortion was legal. That long a drive posed a problem because Amanda's doctors had told her that having lost all her amniotic fluid because her membranes had ruptured, she could develop a severe life-threatening infection at any moment. If that happened while she was driving through the desert of West Texas or sitting in a plane flying to another state, it could be a death sentence.

So Amanda did the only thing she could—wait until she naturally went into labor or until she got so sick her doctors would perform the only medically indicated procedure to treat her condition—an abortion. Three days later, and the day after another Texas abortion ban went into effect, the infection hit Amanda, hard. She developed chills, her temperature spiked, and her blood pressure crashed. When her husband tried talking to her, she wasn't responsive. Amanda's husband rushed her to the hospital, where she was admitted to the labor and delivery unit. At this point, finally, the hospital determined that Amanda's life was enough at risk that they could treat her with the care they should have provided for her days before. They stabilized her enough so that they were able to induce labor without, they now believed, violating Texas's abortion laws. As everyone knew would happen, Willow passed away at delivery.

Amanda's ordeal wasn't over, though. Her initial infection had cleared, but she developed a secondary infection that required three days of treatment in the hospital's intensive-care unit. During this time Amanda was so sick that her family flew in from across the country because they feared it was going to be their last opportunity to see her alive. Thankfully, the treatment of the second infection was successful and Amanda was discharged from the hospital.

However, as a result of this ordeal, Amanda developed such severe scarring from the infection that one of her fallopian tubes is now permanently closed. If Amanda wants to get pregnant again, she has been advised that she will require in vitro fertilization. Moreover, Amanda has described the depression and post-traumatic stress disorder that she suffered for months after this experience as "paralyzing."

In April 2023, Amanda summoned the courage to testify before the United States Senate Judiciary Committee about her experience. Her opening statement concluded,

> What I needed was an abortion, a standard medical procedure. An abortion would have prevented the unnecessary harm and suffering that I endured. Not only the psychological trauma that came with three days of waiting, but the physical harm my body suffered, the extent of which is still being determined. I needed an abortion to protect my life, and to protect the lives of my future babies that I hope and dream I can still have one day. . . . I may have been one of the first who was affected by the overturning of *Roe* in Texas, but I'm certainly not the last. . . . You owe it to me and to Willow and to every other person who may become pregnant in this country to protect our right to safe and accessible healthcare. . . . Being pregnant is difficult and complicated enough. We do not need you to make it even more terrifying and, frankly, downright dangerous to create life in this country. This has gone on long enough.

Along with testifying before the Senate, Amanda joined with other women who were also denied life-saving obstetrical care because of Texas's abortion ban to sue the state of Texas over its law. That suit, filed in early March 2023, was ultimately rejected by the Texas Supreme Court in May 2024,* but the court did acknowledge Amanda's ordeal, saying that it was not what "the law commands."[13]

---

*This is a rapidly changing field. Other than the election update in the epilogue, the material in this book is current through June 2024.

THE NATIONAL LANDSCAPE

As compelling and instructive as these three stories are—of what a child rape victim, a domestic violence survivor, and a woman suffering from a life-threatening condition had to go through to get an abortion after *Dobbs*—they shouldn't eclipse the reality that every abortion seeker's story is unique and that most of them do not involve dire circumstances. Rather, they often involve people who are pregnant who simply no longer want to be—whether the reasons are related to finances, life stage, caring for other children or family members, health complications, maintenance of mental health, wrong partner to raise a child with, or anything else that would lead someone to decide to end their pregnancy.

Ever since *Roe* was overturned, the National Abortion Federation (NAF), the leading professional association of abortion providers, has posted short vignettes on its website, abortionafterroe.com, collected from its abortion hotline. The stories—from people who contacted the hotline either on their own or with the help of a clinic—show the difficulty people had navigating this new environment, even when they receive help from an organization the size of NAF:

- Casey flew from Texas to Colorado to get an abortion once it was illegal in Texas. She made the arrangements for an abortion on her own and paid for her own flight, but when she got to the airport in Colorado, she didn't have any money left in her bank account to pay for the ride to the clinic.
- Maria already had two children when she found out that she was pregnant again. She lived in Louisiana, where abortion became illegal after *Dobbs*, so she drove herself and her two kids to Georgia. Once there, the clinic determined she was further along in her pregnancy than allowable under Georgia law. The best place she could find with an available appointment was in Illinois, so she drove there with her kids to get the care she sought. The extra travel required meals and hotel stays that Maria could not afford on her own.
- Mei lived in Texas and decided to have an abortion when she was six weeks pregnant. Before *Dobbs*, Texas had an abortion ban that limited abortion to before the sixth week of pregnancy, so Mei might have been able to get an abortion in her home state. However, after *Dobbs*, Mei had to travel to New Mexico. As a result, she needed

help paying for her abortion, childcare while she was gone, flights back and forth, a hotel while in New Mexico, rides to and from the airport and clinic, and meals.

All this for quick, simple, safe, and routine medical care.

Each of these stories ends with the person who wanted an abortion being able to get one, albeit through difficult travel and life disruptions that wouldn't have been necessary pre-*Dobbs*. These are the success stories. We also know, though, that there are people who are now unable to get an abortion that they want. Angelica's is one of these stories. She lives in Texas, where she is an undocumented immigrant. Because of *Dobbs*, she couldn't get an abortion in her home state, so she tried finding another option. However, all of the travel possibilities presented to her were too risky. Angelica feared that Texas's internal immigration checkpoints could catch her if she drove to a clinic in another state and that flying would require her to share her identification papers with too many officials. Ultimately, concerned about being deported, Angelica thought it was too risky to travel so she didn't get the abortion she wanted. And the reason she didn't is because of the Supreme Court's decision in *Dobbs*.

DOBBS V. JACKSON WOMEN'S HEALTH ORGANIZATION

When Mississippi's governor Phil Bryant signed a fifteen-week abortion ban on March 19, 2018, everyone knew that the lower federal courts would find it unconstitutional. Some aspects of *Roe v. Wade* and *Planned Parenthood v. Casey* were vague and unclear, but one thing was certain from those opinions: states could not ban abortion before viability of the fetus. Fifteen weeks was roughly two months before viability, so the lower courts, who are bound by Supreme Court precedent, had no choice.

But Governor Bryant didn't sign the law with the intention of winning cases before lower courts; his goal was to make "Mississippi the safest place in America for an unborn child."[15] And in order to do that, he had to take this law to the Supreme Court and convince the justices to change the entirety of United States abortion law.

At the time he signed the bill, achieving that goal looked like an uphill battle. The most recent Supreme Court case on abortion had been *Whole Woman's Health v. Hellerstedt*, the June 2016 case in which a 5–3 majority struck down two Texas abortion restrictions.[16] The justices in the majority applied the precedents of *Roe* and *Casey* without showing any interest in overturning the cases. Almost two years later, when Bryant signed the Mississippi bill, all five of the justices from the majority in *Whole Woman's Health* were still on the Court. President Donald Trump had filled the seat that had been vacant during *Whole Woman's Health* with a conservative, Neil Gorsuch, but Justice Gorsuch replaced another archconservative who had died just before oral argument in the case, Antonin Scalia, and consequently didn't change the balance on the Court with respect to abortion.

But the tide changed on June 27, 2018. That day, just a few hours after the Supreme Court released its last signed opinions of the term, Justice Anthony Kennedy announced his retirement. His retirement letter expressed his appreciation for having had the opportunity to "know, interpret, and defend the Constitution," which, as he saw that duty, included upholding a right to abortion before viability.[17] However, the timing of his retirement called into question his commitment to this particular interpretation of the Constitution: he retired while Donald Trump was president, and Trump had promised during his campaign to nominate people to the Supreme Court who would "automatically" overturn *Roe v. Wade.*

And that's exactly what President Trump did with this opportunity to change the Court's composition. He nominated Brett Kavanaugh, a Federalist Society–backed judge on the federal appeals court for the District of Columbia who had a limited, but clear, history on abortion. He had given a speech in 2017 praising Chief Justice William Rehnquist's jurisprudence, including his dissent in *Roe v. Wade* and his approach to curtailing rights not specified in the Constitution. And later that same year, in his role as a federal appeals judge, Kavanaugh had voted to deny an abortion for an unaccompanied minor who was being held in an immigration detention facility in Texas. Much attention was paid to this issue during Kavanaugh's confirmation hearing, but a long talk with Senator Susan Collins, a pro-choice Republican, convinced her that he would not vote to overturn *Roe*; Collins's vote gave him the votes he needed in the Senate to become a justice and replace Kennedy.

We all know now that Kavanaugh voted to overturn *Roe*, but his appointment alone didn't give the Court the majority it needed to do so. In the 2020 case of *June Medical v. Russo*,[18] Chief Justice John Roberts joined the four liberals on the Court at the time to strike down a Louisiana law that would have shuttered all but one of the state's abortion clinics. Chief Justice Roberts, who had previously been an abortion rights foe, provided the fifth vote in that case based on his sense that he needed to follow precedent, and to him the Louisiana case was almost identical to the 2016 Texas case. This decision meant that as recently as the summer of 2020, there still did not appear to be five votes to overturn *Roe*. President Trump had appointed two conservatives to the Court, both of whom appeared to be reliable votes against the abortion right, but that wasn't enough. And with the presidential election just months away, *Roe* had a fighting chance of surviving the Court's changes.

But *Roe* didn't make it. After surviving many serious health scares over the past two decades, on September 18, 2020, Justice Ruth Bader Ginsburg, a fierce abortion rights defender and one of the necessary votes on the Court to uphold *Roe*, passed away. With only forty-six days to go before the election, President Trump rushed to nominate Amy Coney Barrett, a federal appeals court judge, to replace Justice Ginsburg. Unlike Justice Kavanaugh's record, which some had argued was not enough to know how he truly felt about *Roe*, Barrett's record was undeniable: she was passionately against abortion, had in the past publicly come out in favor of overturning *Roe*, and had consistently voted against abortion rights as a federal judge. After a contentious and rushed process, Barrett was confirmed to the Court just thirty days after her nomination and eight days before the election.

With his third justice confirmed, President Trump had remade the Supreme Court. And Mississippi's fifteen-week ban was perfectly positioned so that Trump's campaign promise about automatically overturning *Roe* could become a reality. Soon after the governor signed the bill, two lower federal courts struck the law down as unconstitutional, as required by *Roe* and *Casey*.[19] At the beginning of the summer of 2020, Mississippi requested that the Supreme Court take the case, and the Court was initially scheduled to consider that request at its private weekly conference on September 29, 2020. With the vacancy created by Justice Ginsburg's death and then Justice Barrett's newly joining the Court, its private discussion of whether to take the case was rescheduled twenty-one times, an unusually high number. Finally, on May 17, 2021, the Court agreed to hear the case.

Mississippi now jumped at the opportunity to ask the Court to overturn *Roe*. In its initial request that the Court take the case, which had occurred when Justice Ginsburg was still alive, Mississippi had *not* asked the Court to overturn *Roe*. Instead, it had sought a ruling that would read *Roe* and *Casey* to allow for pre-viability abortion bans. However, once Justice Ginsburg died and was replaced with Justice Barrett, Mississippi knew how to count to five and went for the gold. In its merits brief in 2021, Mississippi was clear as day: "This Court should overrule *Roe* and *Casey*."

A year later, Mississippi's long game paid off. On June 24, 2022, a five-justice majority of the Supreme Court heeded the state's revised legal plea and overturned *Roe* and *Casey*. Each of the three newly appointed Trump justices voted to overturn the cases, along with the longtime antiabortion stalwarts Justices Clarence Thomas and Samuel Alito. Chief Justice John Roberts also voted to uphold the Mississippi law but, arguing that the Court should only take the drastic step of overturning precedent when it was absolutely required, did not think the Court needed to overturn *Roe* and *Casey* in order to approve the fifteen-week ban.[20] Justices Stephen Breyer, Sonia Sotomayor, and Elena Kagan wrote a joint dissent.

We will save for chapter 1 an in-depth look at the reasoning behind *Dobbs v. Jackson Women's Health Organization*. Important here is what came next. Some states, such as Ohio, had old laws on the books that banned abortion. Because of *Roe*, those laws were not enforceable, but once *Roe* was overruled, these states were free to apply those laws again. Other states had what were called "trigger laws." These laws banned abortion but, because they were passed while *Roe* was still good law, could not immediately take effect. Instead, the laws specifically stated that they would take effect only after *Roe* was overruled. Now that this "trigger" had occurred, these laws took effect. And yet other states passed new laws following the fall of *Roe* now that there was no constitutional impediment to their doing so.

All told, by the end of 2022, six months after *Roe* was overturned, twelve states had bans on abortion at all gestational stages, subject only to very limited and difficult-to-obtain exceptions.[21] These states were Alabama, Arkansas, Idaho, Kentucky, Louisiana, Mississippi, Missouri, Oklahoma, South Dakota, Tennessee, Texas, and West Virginia. Abortion was de facto unavailable in two other states: North Dakota, whose only clinic moved to Minnesota (discussed in more detail in chapter 3), and Wisconsin, where the legal uncertainty about the possibility of enforcement of a nineteenth-century abortion ban ended abortion's availability.

In four other states—Georgia, Florida, Arizona, and Utah—there were now limits on abortion that would not have been constitutional under the *Roe* and *Casey* regime. Georgia banned abortion after six weeks of pregnancy, Florida and Arizona after fifteen weeks, and Utah after eighteen weeks. All of these laws were unconstitutional before *Dobbs* because they banned abortion before viability; after *Dobbs*, the laws could be enforced. Thus, in the immediate aftermath of *Dobbs*, the United States had fourteen states where abortion was completely unavailable and four states where it was time-limited. All because of *Dobbs*.

Notably, however, *Dobbs*'s impact in the second half of 2022 was not monolithically antiabortion. Many states that support abortion rights used *Dobbs* as an impetus to change their law and policy on abortion to increase access. They did this in various ways. Some states took the opportunity to evaluate their abortion laws and remove restrictions that previously limited access. For instance, Illinois and Connecticut expanded the type of medical professionals who can provide abortions for patients. Other states appropriated money to increase access, with Maryland earmarking millions for training abortion providers and New York, Oregon, and California spending tens of millions to improve the state's abortion infrastructure in preparation for an expected increase in people traveling to obtain care. Several states passed a new kind of pro-choice law, an abortion shield law. These laws, pioneered in Connecticut and then expanded upon in Massachusetts and Delaware, protect in-state abortion providers and helpers from being subject to legal action for treating people who travel to those states for abortion care. It is reasonable to observe that none of these changes would have taken place without the looming threat and then ultimate reversal of *Roe*.

The same can be said of *Dobbs*'s impact on the ballot box. Less than six weeks after *Roe* fell, Kansans voted on a ballot initiative that would have ended protection for abortion in the state constitution. Despite the question being on the ballot in a summer primary election when Democrats in the state usually show up in very small numbers, the initiative was defeated by double digits. Three months later, on election day in November, five other states had ballot initiatives related to abortion, and the pro-choice option won in all five. That Vermont and California were among those five states should surprise nobody. Even Michigan might not be that shocking. But the other two states were Montana and Kentucky, showing that, when viewed alongside the Kansas results in August, pro-choice voters can win, even in some of the most conservative states in the country.

Overturning *Roe* also changed the course of the general elections in 2022. Historically, the party that holds the White House suffers major losses in midterm elections. However, almost halfway through Biden's term, Democrats picked up a seat in the Senate and faced minimal losses in the House. Most pundits attributed these historically successful midterm results for the Democrats to the country's views on abortion and the Supreme Court.

HOW *ROE* ENDED, BUT ABORTION DIDN'T

But what changed with abortion provision on the ground is a much more complex story than just recounting the nationwide political trends. Before *Dobbs*, there were over 900,000 abortions in the United States each year.[22] According to the #WeCount study, one of two ongoing studies by public health researchers looking at the impact of *Dobbs* on abortion numbers, in the nine months after *Roe* was overturned over 25,000 people who wanted an abortion were unable to obtain one in the formal medical-care system.[23] That's roughly 3 percent of the number of abortions per year before *Dobbs*.

That there were 25,000 fewer abortions in the formal medical-care system doesn't mean there were 25,000 fewer abortions. An unknown percentage of these people were ultimately able to obtain an abortion thanks to the availability of abortion pills through online pharmacies or informal networks, as well as other forms of self-managed abortion. We don't yet have data to know what that percentage is, and it could be years, if ever, before we do. Until then, we are left knowing that a substantial number of people were unable to get abortions from a clinician in the immediate wake of *Dobbs*, but not knowing what that number is.

However, one of the central questions since *Roe* was overturned is why that number is not higher—in fact, why it isn't much higher. Before *Dobbs*, estimates of the number of people who would not be able to obtain a wanted abortion once states began banning abortion was much higher—ranging from 75,000 to 200,000 per year. By any account, with the data we have so far, *Dobbs* has not had the devastating impact on overall national abortion numbers that many predicted. And, expanding the timeline beyond the immediate months after *Dobbs*, based on data through the beginning of 2024, #WeCount and a separate study from the Guttmacher Institute have both found that, over a year and a half after the decision, *more* abortions are taking place in the United States than before. Indeed, the Guttmacher report found that there were more than one million abortions in the formal health sector in 2023, the highest number in a decade.[24] To put it bluntly, given the dire predictions pre-*Dobbs*, this is shocking.

How exactly people are still getting abortions, even more than before *Dobbs*, is one of the major throughlines of this book. With the overturning of *Roe*, yes, some people lost the ability to obtain an abortion, but so far nowhere near as many as was predicted. That's where this book steps in. In telling the multifaceted stories of what happened in abortion provision the year *Roe* was overturned, we unearth the real story of what happened after *Dobbs*: how *Roe* ended but abortion did not.

As two academics, one in law and the other in sociology, who have studied abortion for decades, we saw the writing on the wall about the end of *Roe*, like almost everyone else who was paying attention. Once the Supreme Court decided to take *Dobbs v. Jackson Women's Health Organization*, there was little doubt in our minds that the Court was very likely to overrule *Roe v. Wade*, and was on the cusp of radically changing abortion law in this country. We were not alone in having this insight, of course. As we talked with abortion providers in our network, we realized their stories were the perfect way to convey the impact of the Supreme Court's changing the fundamental law of abortion. Their stories are the stories of what happens when the Court upends an entire body of law underlying a medical treatment that, before *Dobbs*, nearly one million people had each year. And, as it turns out, their stories show just how abortion has remained a possibility for so many people throughout this country, even as almost a third of states now ban it.

To investigate what was going to happen with the overruling of *Roe*, we spent 2022 repeatedly interviewing people who are deeply involved in the abortion rights world. We chose twenty-four people who worked in different fields in abortion and provided their services in different states and political environments. We interviewed almost all of them three times over the course of 2022: first in early 2022 before *Dobbs* was decided, then again right after the decision was announced, and then a final time six months later, around the end of the year. By talking with each person three times in 2022, we were able to probe with them how clinics, providers, allies, activists, and other abortion rights movement players first anticipated and planned for the Supreme Court ruling, then how they immediately reacted to it, and then ultimately, for most of them, how they were able to continue to serve patients despite the ruling.

Talking to a variety of people at these different moments in 2022 allows us to chronicle what happened on the ground in this important year in abortion rights and to capture just how so many people were still able to get abortions, even after *Roe* was overturned. And, given that we know that abortion numbers have continued to rise after 2022, we can extrapolate from the stories we gathered that year to learn about what has continued to happen through at least the middle of 2024, two years after *Dobbs*.

The different perspectives that explain this phenomenon form the basis of this book's structure. Chapter 1 provides the essential background for the changes the rest of the book covers. It begins with *Roe v. Wade* and then explores the way abortion jurisprudence shifted over the decades but maintained the basic principle that states cannot ban abortion. Under this regime, many states restricted abortion in ways that the Supreme Court allowed; despite some severe restrictions though, abortion remained legal in all fifty states.

What this meant on the ground for people trying to obtain abortions varied across the country. In many states, abortion was already extremely difficult to obtain, especially for people of color, poor people, and people living in rural areas far from an abortion provider. Nonetheless, despite significant variations in abortion availability and accessibility, at a minimum it was legal and available in every state. But abortion opponents pursued a multipronged approach that culminated in 2022's being such a momentous year. Chapter 1 concludes with the abortion battles in Texas and Mississippi, both of which reached the Supreme Court once Justice Barrett was confirmed, with the Mississippi battle providing the antiabortion movement its white whale, the end of *Roe*.

With the stage set, we start the heart of the book with chapter 2, which chronicles the worst of *Dobbs*'s impacts: the closure of abortion clinics or the cessation of the provision of abortion services because of state bans on abortion that would have been unconstitutional during the *Roe* era. This is probably the most predictable outcome of *Dobbs*, and here we introduce three people who struggled through 2022 to move forward in this new reality. Andrea Ferrigno is an abortion clinic administrator from Texas. Andrea began 2022 dealing with the fallout of Senate Bill 8 (SB8), the Texas antiabortion law that authorized bounty hunter lawsuits against any clinic that provided an abortion after the detection of a fetal heartbeat, usually around the sixth week of pregnancy.[25] Just when Andrea and her colleagues figured out a way to continue to provide top-notch care despite SB8, *Dobbs* came along, leaving them no choice but to close their clinics in the state.

This chapter also tells the story of Leah Torres, a doctor in Alabama whose abortion clinic had served a poor, mostly minority population who had difficulty finding any healthcare, not just abortion care, elsewhere in their community. Because of *Dobbs*, Leah and her coworkers had to shut down the clinic's abortion practice. But instead of closing entirely, they pivoted to providing prenatal care and other reproductive health services other than deliveries. In a state that purports to value pregnancy and childbirth so much that it bans abortion, this new endeavor should have been much easier than it has proved to be. The chapter ends by describing the work of Jody Steinauer, a doctor who works to make sure that residents around the country can obtain abortion training. With clinic closures reducing the number of training sites for medical residents, this work is a much more challenging endeavor without the protective umbrella of *Roe*.

But 2022 wasn't all about clinic closures. For some providers, meeting the challenges brought about by *Dobbs* meant being creative in order to continue to see patients. Chapter 3 looks at three different people who, because of the state in which they provided care, were able to explore innovative new options for care even in the post-*Roe* legal setting. For decades, Tammi Kromenaker owned and operated the only abortion clinic in North Dakota. Knowing that her state would be eager to ban abortion once *Roe* was overturned, Tammi secretly purchased and planned the opening of a new clinic across the Red River, in Moorhead, Minnesota. Once the Supreme Court decided *Dobbs*, Tammi moved her clinic to this spot without any interruption in her patients' care.

Moving southwest, Julie Burkhart strategized her response to *Dobbs* by planning to open a new abortion clinic in Wyoming just a month before the Supreme Court was scheduled to rule. Julie's plans were derailed when an antiabortion extremist set fire to her clinic weeks before its planned opening. She wasn't deterred though, continuing her planning while suing the state to prevent implementation of its abortion ban by using a provision of the state constitution originally intended to limit the effects of Obamacare.

Curtis Boyd, a longtime abortion doctor and clinic owner in Texas and New Mexico, was dealing with the two-pronged problem of SB8 in Texas and the upcoming decision from the Supreme Court. To help his patients, he partnered with a pro-choice religious organization to arrange paid-for same-day flights between Texas and New Mexico so patients could get their abortions in New Mexico and return home later that day.

Chapter 4 takes us to three different states that battled legal changes and uncertainty but were ultimately able to keep medical facilities open to serve their patients. In Georgia, Kwajelyn Jackson, the director of a nonprofit clinic, struggled to adapt her services as the state went from being a major hub of care in the South to a state dealing with a new protracted legal battle in state court. This meant changing the care level the clinic provided several times over the course of the second half of 2022. Throughout the constant shifts in care and confusion, Kwajelyn and her colleagues had to care for patients while keeping their eyes on the long-term goal of striking down state restrictions in court and keeping the clinic financially sustainable during the battle.

The story for Karrie Galloway in Utah is similar, but it occurred over a much more concentrated period. Utah's abortion ban took effect almost immediately following *Dobbs*, forcing Karrie to cancel appointments of patients sitting in the waiting room. But then the state courts stepped in to block the state's ban, and Karrie and her colleagues had to quickly pivot to provide care to the people who had been blocked when the ban was in place. The court injunction remained in place for the rest of 2022, but Karrie had to deal with constant attacks in her politically conservative state.

Kelly Flynn dealt with her own uncertainty after *Dobbs*. She owns clinics in Florida and North Carolina, two states where abortion remained legal. However, in both states services changed because of new laws that lowered the state's gestational age limit—the time in pregnancy before which someone can obtain an abortion. So Kelly had to deal with the twin challenge of an influx of patients into both states because of bans in neighboring states while preparing for the possibility of even more restrictions at any moment.

Clinics in states where abortion remained legal and that bordered states where abortion became illegal saw a huge influx in patients and were able to increase their patient volume in response to the crisis of *Dobbs*. Chapter 5 recounts how providers in those states, who knew they were fortunate to remain open and able to care for patients, coped with the surge. The chapter covers the ways that Erin King, a doctor at a southern Illinois clinic that is on the border of Missouri, worked to expand her clinic's services while also assisting patients traveling from all over the South. Likewise, Adrienne Mansanares, the president and CEO of a Planned Parenthood affiliate that covers Colorado, New Mexico, Wyoming, and southern Nevada, saw a staggering increase in patients in each state. The affiliate anticipated this surge, so it strengthened its ability to serve traveling patients by opening a new facility in southern New Mexico, expanding hours of operation, investing in telehealth, and experimenting with new models for delivering abortion care.

Not every state experienced the same surge of travelers as the states that bordered states with bans, but Janet Jacobson, the medical director of a Southern California Planned Parenthood affiliate, and Mercedes Sanchez, an administrator for a series of clinics in Washington State, still had to adapt their services for the new environment. The key for all of these providers was maintaining a high level of care while increasing services. Staffing was a common issue across clinics in the states where abortion remained legal. The chapter ends by considering this issue with additional input from Mary Frank, the director of a program within the National Abortion Federation that performs the crucial work of helping match abortion clinics with staff who can work there.

Perhaps one of the biggest changes in the post-*Roe* landscape, and one of the most significant reasons abortion procedures continue at unexpected levels, is the role of abortion pills. Chapter 6 explores the changed importance of medication abortion, both within the medical system and outside it. Medication abortion had already been the most common form of abortion in the United States for several years before *Dobbs*. The regimen usually involves the use of two drugs in sequence: first mifepristone and then one (and occasionally another) dose of misoprostol, with each misoprostol dose usually consisting of four pills. With abortion now illegal in fourteen states and seriously restricted in several others, abortion providers and advocates understood the power of pills to make abortion more accessible for people who live there, either by traveling to states where abortion remains legal or by using various means to get pills into the states with bans.

Jamie Phifer and Meg Sasse Stern approached this problem by trying to get more pills into people's hands by experimenting within the lawful medical-care delivery model. Jamie is a doctor who, a year before *Dobbs*, opened a telehealth abortion service, Abortion On Demand, that served states where telehealth abortion was legal. When *Dobbs* made abortion illegal in over a dozen states, Jamie had to adapt her service delivery model to try to make it as easy as legally possible for people to obtain pills. Meg works with an abortion provider, Just The Pill, that opened mobile abortion clinics that could be more easily reached by people traveling from states where abortion is banned.

Both Jamie and Meg operated within the framework of the medical establishment, but others were pushing the envelope further in response to the changed environment. Linda Prine, a family physician who also provides abortion care, worked to change the law to allow clinicians in states where abortion remains legal to send pills into states where abortion is banned. Information about her work and those like her is only available because others are getting the word out to the public. Francine Coeytaux is one of the founders of Plan C, a public health campaign that seeks to transform access to abortion in the United States through normalizing the use of abortion pills and increasing access to them. Plan C, which maintains a website to get as much information about abortion pills into the public discourse as possible, had to adapt the site to make sure that the information was helpful in this new legal landscape. It also began to provide information about informal (and legally questionable) means to obtain pills, such as community support networks and mail forwarding. Also recognizing the importance of making sure people know about abortion pills, Amelia Bonow led her organization's efforts to use brash attention-grabbing events and pop culture to inform the public about the option. She also coordinated underground efforts to make sure abortion pills were a known option everywhere in the country.

In this new environment, where abortion's legality and availability are often a function of location, the logistical challenges of moving patients around the country to obtain care and of funding their abortions became a central part of the abortion story. Chapter 7 looks at how abortion funders and travel coordinators, who already had an important job before *Roe* was overturned, tackled this new environment. Oriaku Njoku leads the National Network of Abortion Funds which works with local abortion funds to help fund abortion care and travel. She and her organization became a key part of making sure that patients could access abortion even if they had to travel to other states to do so. Rachel Lachenauer and Chloe Hanson Hebert ran the hotline for the National Abortion Federation. The hotline acted as funder, travel agent, and all-around problem solver for countless abortion seekers, pivoting to serve people in different states trying to surmount different barriers as the landscape quickly shifted after *Dobbs*.

Tackling the most difficult cases, Odile Schalit's organization, the Brigid Alliance, helps patients travel long distance to seek care later in pregnancy. The need for this assistance was already high before *Dobbs* because of the lack of providers who care for patients later in pregnancy. However, after *Dobbs*, the demands on the organization increased drastically. More patients needed to travel long distance to receive care at all stages of pregnancy, and the need for later care also increased as patients were delayed in obtaining an abortion because of local bans. Without the work of the people and organizations highlighted in this chapter, there is no doubt that the number of abortions occurring post-*Dobbs* that the #WeCount and Guttmacher studies have discovered would be much lower.

The changes that *Dobbs* wrought in 2022, chronicled in this book, are just the beginning of the new story of abortion in the United States. So far, that beginning has meant that abortion has continued to be available for most people, although accessing it has often become more disruptive to people's lives. In chapter 8 we speculate on what the future holds: the challenges for people facing medical emergencies to get necessary abortions; the impact of *Dobbs* on general obstetric care; brewing legal battles that could impact ongoing abortion accessibility; and the possible game-changing role of the 2024 elections. Finally, we close by raising the issue that we feel is most central to the future of safe abortion—the sustainability of the extraordinary efforts by providers and allies that occurred in the immediate aftermath of the overthrow of *Roe*.

In explaining throughout this book how abortion has survived the overturning of *Roe*, in no way do we downplay the catastrophic consequences for individuals who have been unable to obtain an abortion because of *Dobbs*. Even with the increase in the number of abortions since *Dobbs*, we know from various sources that many people are still unable to access abortion. And we know, thanks to the landmark Turnaway Study in the 2010s, that people unable to get an abortion they sought are harmed in many ways.[26] Moreover, the lives of people who are now forced to travel and jump through even more hoops to get an abortion are disrupted in significant ways, including an increased risk of health and legal consequences. But perhaps most important, the work required to make abortion possible for all the people who have been disrupted by *Dobbs* is difficult and costly—in time, in money, and in emotion.

But what we have seen so far is that the predicted evisceration of abortion access has not materialized. In fact, because of the people profiled in this book—and many more like them throughout the country—we've seen quite the opposite. In the face of the major blow of overturning *Roe*, abortion has continued, maybe even stronger than before. How people are obtaining and providing abortions is changing and morphing as circumstances require, but people looking for an abortion are, once again, proving that they will always find a way to access it. And providers and supporters, like their predecessors, are proving once more that they will do everything they can to help women and other people capable of pregnancy control this central aspect of their lives.

The Supreme Court hasn't stopped that.

CHAPTER ONE

OVERTURNING *ROE V. WADE*

*The Constitution does not prohibit the citizens of
each State from regulating or prohibiting abortion. Roe
and Casey arrogated that authority. We now overrule
those decisions and return that authority to the people
and their elected representatives.*

—SAMUEL ALITO, US Supreme Court

With these words, Justice Samuel Alito's majority opinion in *Dobbs v. Jackson Women's Health Organization* overturned *Roe v. Wade*, the case that had recognized constitutional protection for the right to abortion.[1] For those in the antiabortion movement, this moment had been nearly fifty years in the making. For those in the abortion rights and justice movement, this moment was exactly what they had feared for decades.

Understanding how we got to this point is the only way to fully appreciate the changes that we cover in the rest of this book. By necessity, the description and analysis offered here is truncated. Doing justice to the endeavor of canvassing the past half century of developments in the law and on the ground reality of abortion would require almost endless space, as each topic constitutes a separate expansive area of study. The goal of this chapter is not to cover the whole field but rather to lay the groundwork necessary to understand both the significance and impact of *Dobbs*.

This chapter will answer many questions. First, what did *Dobbs* overrule? The answer begins with *Roe v. Wade* and then explores the concerted campaign to overrule *Roe* that began almost the day *Roe* was decided. The antiabortion movement successfully chipped away at abortion access but for decades could not accomplish the ultimate goal of overturning *Roe*. As a result, abortion jurisprudence shifted over the decades to allow more restrictions but maintained the basic principle, from *Roe*, that states cannot ban abortion. Under this regime, to the disappointment of the antiabortion movement, abortion remained legal in all fifty states.

With *Roe* the law of the land but state restrictions commonplace, what did this mean for women seeking an abortion? The next part of this chapter will show that, despite abortion's legality, in many states around the country, abortion was extremely difficult to obtain. This challenge was compounded for people of color, poor people, and people living in rural areas far from an abortion provider. For many such women, *Roe* was the law in theory but not in reality. Even so, if they could travel, they could get to a clinic in their state where abortion was legal but highly restricted. Or they could travel to a more liberal state where abortion was both legal and more accessible. Abortion availability and accessibility varied greatly, but at a minimum, it was legal in every state, and providers offering abortion to patients were not at risk of prosecution or losing their license.

Finally, what changed in 2022? The chapter ends by answering that question. Abortion opponents have, since almost the day *Roe* was decided, pursued a multitrack approach that culminated in *Dobbs*. A key part of their approach was to pass legislation that restricted or even outlawed abortion. They passed these laws knowing that the new restrictions would be challenged in court by abortion providers and pro-choice legal organizations. Meanwhile, abortion opponents also worked the political system to create the conditions in which new justices to the Supreme Court would be appointed who would favorably review these laws. This strategy finally bore fruit during the Trump administration: Trump appointed three justices to the Supreme Court, two of whom replaced *Roe*-supportive justices and all of whom were in the Court majority that overturned *Roe*.

The combined strategy struck gold when the laws of Texas and Mississippi came before the newly constituted Court. Texas's passage of SB8, the ban on abortion after six weeks of pregnancy, led, in late 2021, to the Supreme Court giving its first indication what the newest justices thought of the right to abortion. Then, when faced with the Mississippi law banning abortion after fifteen weeks, the Court took the step antiabortion activists had been dreaming of, finally overruling *Roe v. Wade*. That opinion paved the way for the experiences chronicled in the rest of the book.

ROE V. WADE

Justice Harry Blackmun, the lead author of *Roe v. Wade*, thought he had solved the problem of abortion, possibly once and for all. In the 1973 opinion, he could have written that the Texas law at issue in the case—a complete ban on abortion with minimal exceptions—was unconstitutional and stopped there. Instead, he added a section to the opinion creating the trimester framework: in the first trimester of pregnancy, states could not regulate abortion; in the second trimester, states could regulate the procedure but only to further the health of the pregnant woman; and in the third trimester, states could ban abortion but had to have exceptions for the health and life of the woman. This kind of detailed, forward-looking guidance to state legislatures is unusual in a Supreme Court opinion, but Justice Blackmun believed that by being this specific, states would know what they could and couldn't do, and the Court might never again have to confront the issue.

He was wrong. Stupendously wrong. Rather than ending the matter with respect to constitutional litigation, *Roe v. Wade* kicked off five decades of a seemingly endless back-and-forth between state legislatures and the federal courts. And all of it was focused on interpreting and attacking Justice Blackmun's original reasoning and words.

So, what did he say in *Roe*? It's a long opinion that covers a lot of ground, but boiled down, there are four important parts of *Roe* that drove the conclusion and then what came after. First, Justice Blackmun surveyed history to show "that the restrictive criminal abortion laws in effect in a majority of States today are of relatively recent vintage."[2] He recognized that then-recent American history included bans on abortion in every state, but at the time of the founding through the first half of the 1800s, if abortion was banned, it was banned only after quickening, the point during a pregnancy when fetal movement could first be felt. He also surveyed history from English common and statutory law to medical ethics as well as modern medical association statements to conclude that abortion was also not a disfavored practice throughout history. This historical look at abortion helped set the stage for the legal analysis that followed.

Next, Justice Blackmun tackled the legal framework for the case. In doing so, he looked at the history of a legal doctrine called substantive due process. This doctrine is rooted in the Fourteenth Amendment's Due Process Clause, which states, "Nor shall any state deprive any person of life, liberty, or property without due process of law."[3] The key words here are "liberty" and "due process." Dating back to the early 1900s, the Supreme Court had interpreted the word "liberty" to include various rights that are not listed in the Constitution. If the Court determined a right was protected under the concept of "liberty," then a state could not deprive someone of that right without a strong reason for doing so. Otherwise, the state would be acting arbitrarily, and that would constitute a denial of due process.

This is where the key step in *Roe* happened. The Court found that the right to terminate a pregnancy was one of the rights included in the concept of "liberty." Justice Blackmun's opinion reached that conclusion on the basis of two lines of thinking. First he looked at the precedent that had found other rights protected under the idea of liberty. Those cases had to do with child-rearing, contraception, marriage, and procreation. To Justice Blackmun and the Court majority, the right to terminate a pregnancy naturally fit within the same broader concept of decisional and personal autonomy that formed the basis of these other rights. Second, Justice Blackmun looked at the importance that the right to an abortion had in women's lives. Overall, he said that the "detriment that the State would impose upon the pregnant woman by denying this choice altogether is apparent."[4]

Because the right to terminate a pregnancy is included in the concept of "liberty," the Court explained that any restriction on it would be subject to "strict scrutiny." This term means that a state can restrict that right only if it has a compelling reason to do so and even then, does so in the least restrictive way possible. This concept of strict scrutiny is commonly applied for protected rights under the Due Process Clause as well as other parts of the Constitution.

Third, Justice Blackmun's opinion addressed the ongoing dispute as to whether a fetus is a person. The opinion did not answer this question as a general matter. Rather, Justice Blackmun wrote that people are, of course, free to believe what they want on the basis of their own sense of morality, ethics, religion, science, and whatever else contributes to an individual's answer to this question. It is not for the Court, he said, to "speculate as to the answer" to this difficult question.[5] However, the Court is responsible for answering whether, under the Constitution, a fetus is a person. That question is something within the Court's capacity to decide, and here the Court decided that it was not. In light of how the Constitution uses the word "person" in other contexts, the Court concluded it would make no sense to consider a fetus a person. Moreover, other areas of law, both federal and state, had not used "person" to include fetuses. Thus, on this thorny issue of American politics, the opinion in *Roe* said that under the Constitution, a fetus is not a person.

Finally, in applying strict scrutiny to the abortion ban, *Roe* clarified which state interests were sufficient to restrict the right. The Court recognized that states have an interest in the health of the person who is pregnant as well as in the potential life of the fetus.

The key to the Court's particular conclusion about both the Texas law and the trimester framework is that those interests progress over time during a pregnancy. In the first trimester, abortion is safe—indeed, safer than childbirth (as is true in the second and third trimesters as well)—and the fetus cannot survive outside the womb, so the state's interests in health and potential life are not compelling enough to justify a ban on abortion. In the second trimester, the procedure is, according to the Court, riskier, so the state's interest in health is compelling, but the fetus still cannot survive outside the woman. Thus, the state can regulate the procedure to protect the woman's health but cannot ban the procedure outright. In the third trimester, the interest in potential life is now compelling because viability is, by definition, the point at which the fetus can survive outside the woman. But the state still has to protect the health and life of the pregnant woman, so the state can ban abortion but must provide exceptions in case the pregnancy threatens her health or life.

As controversial as *Roe* became in American law and history, it was not a closely divided opinion at the Court. There were only two dissenting votes, from Justices Byron White and William Rehnquist. Their dissents focused on the interpretation of precedent and history. They argued that the cases that Justice Blackmun relied upon were not expansive enough to cover abortion and that the historical record shows more regulation of abortion than Justice Blackmun indicated. In particular, Justice Rehnquist argued that most states banned abortion at the time of the Fourteenth Amendment's ratification in 1868, which should mean, he claimed, that the Fourteenth Amendment does not prohibit states from banning abortion in 1973.

In both *Roe* and another abortion case decided the same day out of Georgia, *Doe v. Bolton*, the makeup of the majority and dissenting voting blocs on the Court indicated that the constitutionality of abortion bans was not as polarizing as it became after *Roe*.[6] Both the majority and the dissent in both cases consisted of justices who were appointed by both parties. In the majority were five justices appointed by Republican presidents (including *Roe's* author, Justice Blackmun) and two appointed by Democratic presidents. In dissent, Justice White was appointed by a Democrat and Justice Rehnquist by a Republican. This is a stark difference from the makeup of the *Dobbs* voting blocs.

With the decision in *Roe*, abortion delivery instantaneously changed in this country. Prior to *Roe*, abortion had been illegal for decades in every state in the country. Immediately prior to *Roe*, four states had legalized abortion—New York, Washington, Hawaii, and Alaska. Thirteen other states had begun liberalizing their abortion laws by increasing the scope of the exceptions in which abortion was allowed beyond a threat to the woman's life. But in the rest of the country, abortion was illegal in almost all circumstances.

As soon as *Roe* was decided, abortion became legal up to viability (or beyond) in all states. In some parts of the country, activists who had been providing abortions clandestinely or helping patients travel to states where abortion was legal quickly began operating abortion clinics where this had previously been banned. In other locations, hospitals filled the gap because of practical barriers to opening stand-alone clinics. By the numbers, *Roe's* impact was drastic. In 1975, over one million legal abortions were performed in the country, and by 1980, over 1.5 million.

The procedure became much safer, too, as the mortality rate due to abortion dropped from between 60 to 80 per 100,000 cases before *Roe* to just 1.3 afterwards. Abortion was not accessible everywhere, though, as most providers were concentrated in metropolitan areas; women seeking abortion in rural states had to travel to have the procedure.[7]

FROM *ROE* TO *CASEY*

Even though abortion was now legal everywhere and service delivery was expanding in these new ways, antiabortion legislators were not dissuaded by *Roe*. In Missouri, for instance, just over a year after *Roe* was decided, the legislature passed a comprehensive abortion bill that, among other things, required a woman obtaining an abortion to get the consent of her husband, required a minor to get the consent of a parent, required the physician to try to preserve the life of the fetus during the procedure, and prohibited the most common form of second-trimester abortion at the time. Other states, such as Pennsylvania and Massachusetts, did the same.[8]

Perhaps the post-*Roe* abortion law with the broadest impact came from the federal government. For the first few years after *Roe* was decided,

Medicaid covered abortions for indigent women. This coverage resulted in almost 300,000 abortions funded by the program each year.[9] Antiabortion members of Congress did not approve. The leading voice was that of Henry Hyde, a House Republican from Illinois. He recognized that Congress could not end legal abortion because it could not overrule the Supreme Court, so he devised a strategy that, he believed, would be the next best thing: he would make it impossible for poor women to use government medical assistance to pay for the procedure. And he supported his plan by using the worst of racialized code language: "I certainly would like to prevent, if I could legally, anybody having an abortion, a rich woman, a middle-class woman, or a poor woman. Unfortunately, the only vehicle available is the [Medicaid] bill. A life is a life. The life of a little ghetto kid is just as important as the life of a rich person. And so we proceed in this bill."[10] The so-called Hyde Amendment, which barred the use of federal Medicaid funds for the provision of abortion, passed as a budget rider in 1976 and has been approved by Congress every year since then.

These and other new restrictions on abortion served multiple functions. Primarily they were attempts to restrict abortion. If the restrictions were left in place, the antiabortion movement hoped they would reduce the number of abortions. However, there was a separate goal here, as these restrictions were an essential part of the antiabortion movement's multifaceted strategy to overturn *Roe*. The Supreme Court only decides cases that are appealed to it; it can't reach out and decide issues proactively. Thus, if the movement's ultimate goal was for the Court to overturn *Roe*, it needed cases in the court system that would work their way up to the Supreme Court for it to decide. These new abortion restrictions were the vehicle. The abortion rights movement was certain to challenge these laws in court, and those challenges could eventually make their way to the Supreme Court.

The antiabortion movement was right, as each of the restrictions mentioned was challenged and made its way to the Supreme Court. In the first decade after *Roe*, though, the movement was met with a Court that was mostly hostile to abortion restrictions. It struck down the most onerous restrictions out of Missouri, Pennsylvania, and Massachusetts, prohibiting the requirement of spousal consent for married women, restrictions on common procedures, two-parent consent requirements for minors, and laws that required providers to preserve the life of the fetus during an abortion.[11]

However, in a major win for the antiabortion movement, the Supreme Court allowed restrictions on both state and federal public funding for abortion. In both 1977 and 1980, the Court reasoned that *Roe* was based on privacy, the notion that the government can't take measures to interfere with the abortion decision. Whether the government uses public dollars to fund an abortion is not, the Court reasoned, about privacy. Rather, the Court said, people can still make the private choice to have an abortion and if they don't have enough money to pay for it, that is not because the government interfered but rather because of their own life circumstances. Justices Thurgood Marshall and William Brennan dissented, saying that the right to abortion is meaningless for poor women who don't have the means to pay for it, but the majority was unmoved. *Roe* required the government not to interfere with the right to abortion; it did not require the government to affirmatively assist people in exercising the right.[12]

Getting the Supreme Court's blessing on the Hyde Amendment was a victory for the antiabortion movement, but they wanted more. Over the next decade, the movement worked in conjunction with the wider conservative legal movement on two goals: theorizing and promoting originalism as a method of interpreting the Constitution; and appointing new justices to the Supreme Court who were skeptical of or outright hostile to *Roe*. Simultaneously, other aspects of the anti-*Roe* strategy moved in parallel with these legal maneuvers focused on the Supreme Court: capturing the Republican Party, making actual abortion access difficult through overregulation, engaging in violence and harassment against abortion providers and clinics, marginalizing abortion care within the medical community, and stigmatizing the procedure and those who have it in popular discourse. These efforts worked alongside the movement's efforts that were more directly focused on the Supreme Court.

But the rise of originalism and major shifts at the Supreme Court had the most direct impact on the future of *Roe*. Originalism is a theory of how to interpret the Constitution that states that the meaning of constitutional provisions is fixed at the time the provision was ratified. Thus, the meaning of the Fourteenth Amendment, added to the Constitution in 1868, was fixed in 1868, and societal changes that occurred after then are irrelevant to the provision's meaning. From the 1970s to the 1980s, originalism grew in importance among legal conservatives. In 1985, United States Solicitor General Charles Fried used originalism to argue before the Supreme Court, for the first time on behalf of the United States, that

Roe should be overruled. In the United States' brief to the Court in a case challenging Pennsylvania's newest antiabortion law, Fried argued that *Roe* had no "moorings" in the "framers' intention."[13]

Originalism was becoming more a part of constitutional interpretation discourse but needed judicial proponents to really make a difference in the law. Justice William Rehnquist had made an originalist argument in his dissent in *Roe*, but it wasn't until the rapid transformation of the Court's makeup under Presidents Reagan and Bush that originalism found its most ardent proponents among the justices. Over the rest of the 1970s, there was only one new justice on the Court, when President Ford replaced Justice William Douglas with John Paul Stevens. Although Douglas, who was in the *Roe* majority, had been appointed by a Democrat and Stevens by a Republican, this change did not alter the balance on abortion rights, as Justice Stevens was a reliable vote in favor of abortion rights throughout his almost thirty-five-year career on the Court.

The real changes relating to abortion (and many other issues) came in the 1980s. The first change came in 1981, when Justice Potter Stewart, also in the *Roe* majority, was replaced by a conservative, Sandra Day O'Connor. Much attention was paid to her nomination as someone who would vote to overturn *Roe*. And while she was very skeptical of *Roe* in her first decade on the Court, she ultimately voted in *Planned Parenthood v. Casey* to uphold the basic holding of *Roe*, that states cannot make abortion illegal.

Two other appointments during this era, Justices Anthony Kennedy and David Souter, also failed to alter the balance on *Roe*. Justice Kennedy, nominated by President Reagan and confirmed in 1988, replaced Lewis Powell, another member of the *Roe* majority. Although Justice Kennedy often voted to uphold abortion restrictions, he ultimately voted with Justice O'Connor to reaffirm *Roe*. Justice David Souter was another Republican appointee from this era. Nominated by President Bush and joining the Court in 1990, he replaced William Brennan, one of the Court's most vocal liberals and another vote in the majority in *Roe*. These three new justices—O'Connor, Kennedy, and Souter—all appointed by Republicans and all replacing members of the *Roe* majority, shifted the Court in a more conservative direction in many ways, even on abortion restrictions, but they were not opposed to *Roe* entirely, nor were they reliable originalists.

The truly consequential changes on the Court came with the appointments of Antonin Scalia and Clarence Thomas. Both justices were vocal critics of *Roe* as well as strong proponents and proselytizers of originalism.

In 1986, Justice Scalia joined the Court when Justice Rehnquist became the chief justice, replacing Chief Justice Warren Burger, who had been in the *Roe* majority. Justice Scalia served on the Court for twenty-nine years and during that time never voted to strike down an abortion restriction and almost always wrote separate opinions attacking *Roe* and urging that it be overturned.

The appointment of Justice Clarence Thomas rounds out this era, as he replaced Justice Thurgood Marshall in 1991. Marshall, another member of the *Roe* majority, had been a stalwart liberal and strong supporter of *Roe*, and his replacement by one of the most conservative members the Court has seen in modern times was a major shift. Justice Thomas, like Justice Scalia, has never voted to strike down an abortion restriction, was a consistent critic of *Roe*, and ultimately joined the majority in *Dobbs*.

Justices Scalia and Thomas were important additions to the Court not only because of their reliable opinions against *Roe* but also because they became the two most prominent voices of originalism in American law. With their ascension to the Court, originalism moved into a much more high-profile position. Over the course of their time on the bench (with Justice Thomas's still ongoing), they were effective in moving the Court, the academy, and American legal thinking in general in the direction of originalism, something that we continue to see evidence of today as the Court regularly churns out purportedly originalist analysis to support its constitutional decisions.

PLANNED PARENTHOOD V. CASEY

By 1992, less than two decades after *Roe*, the Court had been remade. *Roe*'s two dissenters—Justices White and Rehnquist—remained on the Court, but only Justice Blackmun, the author of *Roe*, remained from the majority in that case. All six of the other justices who were in the *Roe* majority had been replaced by justices nominated by a Republican president—five of them having been nominated at a time when overturning *Roe* had become a central focus of Supreme Court nominations. After all these changes it was difficult to see *Roe* surviving much longer.

The writing on the wall had been quite clear just a few years prior. In 1989, the Court decided a case out of Missouri, *Webster v. Reproductive Health Services*, that dealt with another cluster of Missouri abortion restrictions, all of which the Court upheld.[14] In the Court's 5–4 decision, four of the five justices in the majority gave strong indication that they would overrule *Roe*.

The fifth justice in the majority, Justice O'Connor, showed a bit of moderation. She argued that the Missouri regulations could be upheld by narrowing *Roe* rather than overturning it. She suggested applying what she termed the "undue burden" test, which is a more relaxed standard than *Roe*'s "strict scrutiny" test, but not as relaxed as the others in the majority wanted. With five justices now arguing to overrule or modify *Roe*, Justice Blackmun's dissent sounded a warning about the future of *Roe*, saying he "fear[ed] for the future" of abortion rights.[15]

When *Planned Parenthood of Southeastern Pennsylvania v. Casey* came to the Court three years later, the same five justices who had been in the *Webster* majority were now joined by two additional Republican appointees, Justices Thomas and Souter. As a result, many people among both Court observers and the general public feared that *Casey* spelled the end of *Roe*. However, despite the numbers being against *Roe*, it survived, at least in part.

Even before *Casey*, the Supreme Court had developed some expertise with Pennsylvania abortion restrictions.[16] In 1979, in *Colautti v. Franklin*, the Court had struck down many Pennsylvania provisions for being too vague to give doctors clear guidance as to what the law requires. The Pennsylvania legislature was not deterred and passed new abortion restrictions in response. That law was then struck down by the Supreme Court in 1986 in *Thornburgh v. American College of Obstetricians and Gynecologists*. Still not dissuaded, in 1988 the Pennsylvania legislature passed yet more amendments to their Abortion Control Act. These new provisions became the basis of *Planned Parenthood v. Casey*.

At issue in the case were six different aspects of Pennsylvania law: a requirement that married women notify their spouse before they had an abortion; a requirement that minors get the consent of one parent or go before a judge for permission; a requirement that everyone go through an informed consent process above and beyond any other medical procedure; a requirement that everyone wait twenty-four hours after initially contacting the abortion provider before having the procedure; a narrow definition of "medical emergency" to permit bypassing the statute's requirements; and a reporting requirement for abortion facilities. The federal appeals court that covers Pennsylvania had upheld all parts of the law other than the spousal notification provision. Samuel Alito, the future author of *Dobbs*, was a judge on this court at the time and was part of the panel that decided this case. He wrote a separate opinion arguing that *all* parts of the Pennsylvania law were constitutional, including the spousal notification provision.

On appeal to the Supreme Court, both sides turned a case about specific provisions of Pennsylvania law into a case about *Roe v. Wade*.[17] The appeals court had conducted a deep dive into the various recent Supreme Court rulings on abortion and, although it had no authority to overrule Supreme Court precedent, concluded that the proper way to analyze abortion restrictions was not through *Roe*'s strict scrutiny test but rather through the undue burden test developed in Justice O'Connor's separate writings in *Webster* and other abortion cases.

Only the lawyer for Pennsylvania defended this analysis before the Supreme Court, but his arguments were overshadowed by the other advocates in court that day. Kathryn Kolbert, the lawyer for the abortion clinics challenging Pennsylvania's law, focused more on the abstract issue of the standard of review rather than the specific abortion restrictions at issue in the case. In doing so, she urged the justices to reaffirm *Roe* and hold that the strict scrutiny test still applied in abortion cases. "To abandon strict scrutiny for a less protective standard," she told the justices, "would be the same as overruling *Roe*." Arguing the exact opposite, the solicitor general of the United States argued that the correct analysis would be to broadly allow states to regulate abortion.[18]

At a press conference following oral argument, Kolbert was not optimistic. "It is my expectation the Court will abandon abortion as a fundamental right," she said candidly.[19] And when the decision was released two months after argument, she was right—the Court had abandoned the language of fundamental rights and the strict scrutiny test that accompanied it. But what it replaced that test with and how it did that was complicated.

The Court's nine justices fractured into three different camps that mirrored the advocates who argued the case. Two justices—*Roe*'s author, Blackmun, along with Stevens—argued that the Court should continue the analysis from *Roe* and that most (Stevens) or all (Blackmun) of Pennsylvania's provisions were unconstitutional. On the opposite end of the spectrum, four justices—*Roe*'s original dissenters, Rehnquist and White, along with the newcomer originalists Scalia and Thomas—would have overturned *Roe* and given states broad leeway to regulate or even ban abortion.

That left three justices who decided the outcome of the case—Justices O'Connor, Kennedy, and Souter. These three justices, none of whom had been on the Court for *Roe*, adopted a compromise position that claimed to uphold "the essential holding of *Roe*" while also changing the standard of review to the "undue burden" test Justice O'Connor had championed in previous abortion cases. They tried to give a clear explanation of what this test meant: "An undue burden exists, and therefore a provision of law is invalid, if its purpose or effect is to place a substantial obstacle in the path of a woman seeking an abortion before the fetus attains viability."[20]

The justices went on to discuss what they called "guiding principles" for the undue burden analysis. They said that states are allowed to "create a structural mechanism" to "express profound respect for the life of the unborn." As long as these laws don't create a "substantial obstacle" for the exercise of the right to choose, states can try to persuade women "to choose childbirth over abortion" and impose requirements "designed to foster the health of a woman seeking an abortion."[21]

Notable here is what the justices jettisoned from *Roe*. Although they said they were upholding the "essential holding" of *Roe*, gone was the notion that abortion was a fundamental right, that the proper standard was strict scrutiny, and that courts should analyze restrictions differently during pregnancy's different trimesters. Instead, what these justices said mattered in *Roe*, and what they carried forward in *Casey*, is that states cannot ban abortion until after viability. But before viability, states can enact restrictions that are burdensome and amount to obstacles as long as those restrictions aren't too burdensome and don't create too much of an obstacle.

How these justices applied this new standard to Pennsylvania's abortion law shows why the clinics urged the Court to apply strict scrutiny. Under the new undue burden test, the three justices reached the same result as the lower court: all of Pennsylvania's provisions were constitutional except for the requirement that women notify their husbands. They did not believe, for instance, that minors being required to talk with a parent or appear before a judge or rural women being required to make two trips to a clinic and wait twenty-four hours in between visits was too burdensome. Rather, these provisions, like the others at issue in the case besides the spousal notification requirement, were legitimate ways for Pennsylvania to express its respect for potential life. Under Court customs for counting votes, these three justices' votes were combined with those of the four justices who would have overturned *Roe* in its entirety to create a Court majority allowing almost all of Pennsylvania's restrictions to go into effect.

THE ABORTION OBSTACLE COURSE

Casey was an obvious compromise. Abortion could not be banned, but it could be regulated, sometimes in very restrictive ways. And sure enough, antiabortion states heeded this call. As we detailed in our previous book, *Obstacle Course: The Everyday Struggle to Get an Abortion in America*, what emerged after *Casey* was a national landscape where abortion access varied dramatically.[22] Until *Dobbs*, there was no place in the country where abortion was banned. However, on the way from *Casey* to *Dobbs*, antiabortion legislators became increasingly creative and aggressive in regulating abortion in ways that made it very difficult for some people in some locations to get the care they sought.

Because the restrictions varied from state to state, there was no one pre-*Dobbs* path to getting an abortion. However, even with *Roe* in place, abortion restrictions in many states impacted every step in the process of how someone obtained an abortion, from the decision-making through the abortion itself. Looking at each step in the process shows just how difficult antiabortion state legislatures made it for women to obtain an abortion.

DECISION-MAKING: Most women choosing an abortion are certain of their decision and do so for reasons connected to their own personal life. However, under the *Casey* regime, states took creative approaches to pushing women to not choose abortion. For instance, they insulated medical providers from lawsuits when they gave incorrect information to patients to make them less likely to have an abortion, prohibited abortion referrals in some circumstances, and allowed fake antiabortion clinics to lie and deceive women who consulted them when considering an abortion. States also prohibited women from basing their abortion decision on certain reasons such as the sex or chromosomal analysis of the fetus and made minors consult with either a parent or a judge in making their decision. All of this was geared toward overriding people's decisions to terminate their pregnancies.

FINDING AND GETTING TO A CLINIC: Abortion providers had been dwindling in number for a long time before *Roe* was overturned owing to a variety of factors (such as increasing regulation of abortion facilities) that made it difficult to operate, harassment and violence against abortion providers, and a steady decline in the number of abortions nationwide. As a result, in 2020, 89 percent of counties in the United States did not have a known abortion provider and six or seven states had only one abortion clinic.[23] This meant that many people seeking an abortion were forced to travel long distances to see a provider. For some, travel is easy. But for many people, especially the majority of abortion patients, who are indigent, travel posed great difficulty and could even be a complete barrier.[24]

PAYING FOR THE ABORTION: Compared to the cost of American healthcare in general, abortion is not expensive. However, because 75 percent of abortion patients are at or below 200 percent of the poverty line, this low-cost medical care can be very difficult for many to afford. Private or public insurance should cover the cost. However, not everyone has medical insurance. Furthermore, many states banned insurance from covering abortion, and the Hyde Amendment prohibits federal Medicaid dollars from paying for an abortion. Two-thirds of states followed suit for state Medicaid dollars. As a result, those who cannot afford the cost of their abortion are faced with the no-win choice public health insurance was designed to cure: choosing to pay for their healthcare or choosing to pay for other necessities in life such as food, clothing, shelter, and utility bills. The best estimates are that about one-quarter of women who would have otherwise chosen to have an abortion were unable to because of the Medicaid coverage ban.

GETTING INSIDE THE CLINIC: Getting into a medical facility is something most people don't think twice about once they've found the building. However, for abortion patients, getting inside can be like crossing a battle zone. Antiabortion extremists have developed many tactics to make it difficult to get inside, from mass protests and parades to hostile confrontations and prayer sessions that disrupt clinic access. Clinics employ volunteer escorts and rearrange their physical location to try to reduce the impact of the antiabortion presence. In most places in the country they are left with very little recourse under the law. The Supreme Court had already, pre-*Dobbs*, made it difficult to keep the peace by creating any kind of buffer or bubble zone around a clinic. As a result, antiabortion protesters are often able to position themselves right in front of the clinic entrance so they have direct access to patients coming and going.

COUNSELING: The abortion counseling process is one that is individualized to each patient. However, antiabortion states had inserted themselves into the counseling process in various ways, establishing requirements that are not a part of any other form of medicine and that do not help the patient. For instance, some states required abortion providers to give patients written information about abortion that was deceptive or incorrect; to tell patients that their fetus could feel pain, despite a lack of scientific evidence to support that claim; to inform patients about risks of abortion that are not supported by evidence; to advise patients that a medication abortion can be reversed (which is not medically accurate); and to perform ultrasounds and describe the results even when it was not medically necessary to do so. Almost all of these requirements had been allowed by various federal courts, including some at the Supreme Court.

WAITING PERIODS: Most people are used to waiting to get a medical appointment or have a procedure. However, those waits are based on the availability of the medical care provider. For abortion patients, providers have mastered keeping their schedules open because of the time-sensitive nature of the care. Yet state legislatures have passed laws that require patients to wait an extra amount of time beyond what providers might require to accommodate their own schedules, and the Supreme Court has allowed these. These waiting periods started at twenty-four hours but then, in some states, stretched to forty-eight hours or even seventy-two hours. Waiting three days doesn't sound like that much, but when states require in-person visits for the first and second appointments, it can mean multiple long trips for patients who might not have the flexibility in their schedules.

THE ABORTION: Rather than defer to the medical expertise of the trained professionals involved in abortion care, antiabortion legislators insisted they knew better and told the professionals how to provide care. They limited how providers could use telehealth in conjunction with medication abortion. They prohibited certain procedures from being used to perform the abortion. They restricted which medical personnel could perform the abortion. They prohibited abortion at twenty weeks of pregnancy, which is several weeks before viability. And they made it difficult for hospital providers to care for abortion patients.

———————

These restrictions, when looked at together, show the limitations of the *Casey* regime. No state had an active abortion ban, but many states piled restriction upon restriction to make actual access to abortion difficult for many and nearly impossible for some. For the most part, courts hearing challenges to these laws did not consider them to be unduly burdensome or the obstacles substantial. Those who felt these restrictions the most were women of color or women who were poor or rural, but the difficulties such individuals faced were mostly ignored by the privileged judges who reviewed their claims. As long as clinics were able to stay open and abortion remained legal, the courts allowed states to put hurdles in place that made care difficult to access.

This regime lasted for thirty years, from *Casey* in 1992 to *Dobbs* in 2022. However, no one was really happy with this resolution. Abortion rights supporters frequently claimed that while abortion was legal in theory, in practice it was inaccessible for too many. Abortion opponents celebrated making abortion more difficult to access but viewed these restrictions as falling short of their true goal of overturning *Roe* so they could make abortion illegal, not just difficult to obtain.

THE RUN-UP TO *DOBBS*

Because of that dissatisfaction with merely being able to heavily regulate abortion, the effort to overturn *Roe* never fully abated. In the three decades after *Casey*, originalism continued its ascendancy within the courts and in academia. During the same time period, Republican presidents nominated and appointed five new justices to the Supreme Court (Chief Justice Roberts and Justices Alito, Gorsuch, Kavanaugh, and Barrett) while Democratic presidents nominated and appointed only four (Justices Ginsburg, Breyer, Sotomayor, and Kagan). Importantly, three of the Republican appointees replaced justices who had supported abortion rights—Alito replaced O'Connor, Kavanaugh replaced Kennedy, and Barrett replaced Ginsburg (although Ginsburg had replaced White, who was an original *Roe* dissenter). These changes gave the Court a decidedly 6–3 Republican edge by the end of 2020.

This new Court quickly had the opportunity to show the world how it viewed abortion. Antiabortion states had been pushing the envelope with more burdensome restrictions, in particular with restrictions that lowered the gestational age limit. Mississippi's fifteen-week ban, passed in 2018, was one such law. As discussed earlier, this ban had been struck down by the lower courts that reviewed it, even the notoriously conservative and antiabortion Fifth Circuit Court of Appeals. But Mississippi did not give up and had already asked the Supreme Court to hear the case by the time

Justice Barrett was confirmed. Eventually, in May 2021, the Court agreed to do so, setting the stage for a major battle over the future of *Roe*.

However, while the briefs were being written in that case and before it was argued, a surprise abortion case came before the Court, one that gave the public a hint of how the newly constituted Court would treat *Roe*. The case came from Texas, which in the spring of 2021 passed a unique law, Senate Bill 8, which banned abortion at six weeks but did so in a novel way. Rather than enforce the ban with criminal penalties, monetary fines, or licensure consequences, SB8 enforced the ban by allowing anyone to sue to enforce the law. There was no requirement that the person bringing the lawsuit have any connection to the person getting an abortion or the person providing the abortion. And the person bringing the lawsuit could sue not only the abortion provider but anyone who aided or abetted the abortion, including those who funded it. In effect it was enforcement by bounty.

Texas's abortion clinics challenged the law shortly before it was to take effect, on September 1, 2021. The federal district court initially sided with the abortion providers, but the Fifth Circuit Court of Appeals ruled that the district court's order should be put on hold, which would allow SB8 to go into effect four days later. The clinics filed an emergency appeal with the Supreme Court two days before the law was to take effect, arguing that if the Court did not act immediately, all of the clinics in Texas would have to stop abortions after six weeks, thus drastically harming the women of Texas and denying them their constitutional right to pre-viability abortions.

The Supreme Court, in its first ruling on abortion with Justice Barrett and without Justice Ginsburg, wasn't moved. The Court did not issue a decision before the calendar turned from August 31 to September 1, remaining silent and thus allowing the law to take effect. When the Court did finally rule, it issued a short unsigned order saying that, although the clinics raised "serious questions," they had not convinced a majority of the justices on the "complex and novel" procedural questions raised by SB8's bounty-enforcement scheme.[25] Four justices—Chief Justice Roberts and Justices Breyer, Sotomayor, and Kagan—dissented, arguing that it was important to block the law so the courts could fully consider what Justice Sotomayor called a "flagrantly unconstitutional law engineered to prohibit women from exercising their constitutional rights."[26]

Abortion clinics in Texas scrambled to deal with the new situation. They stopped performing abortions after six weeks, which in pregnancy math (which counts the first day of the start of a woman's last menstrual period as the first day of pregnancy) is only two weeks after someone notices they missed their period. Clinics worked with nonprofit logistical and financial support agencies to care for patients as quickly as possible if they could be seen before the six-week mark or, if not, to transport them out of state. Many more women than anticipated were still able to get abortions, even with SB8 in place, but many were not. Thanks to the Supreme Court's showing no concern about this devastating impact, SB8 had its desired effect.

The legal wrangling over SB8 was not over, though. The clinics continued their case in the lower courts over the next several weeks and then once again asked the Supreme Court to hear the case. With SB8 in place, the Court took the case challenging it and heard oral argument on an expedited basis on November 1. In *Whole Woman's Health v. Jackson*, the Court ruled a month later (nine days after *Dobbs* was argued) that the lawsuit could go forward but only against the state's abortion provider licensing officials and only if they actually had authority to implement some part of SB8. The Court left SB8 in effect while the lawsuit continued in the lower courts, once again showing no concern that the then-still-existing constitutional right to abortion was being curtailed in Texas. When the Texas Supreme Court ruled in March 2022 that the licensing officials did not in fact, under Texas law, have any SB8 enforcement authority, the federal lawsuit was over.[27]

All in all, the newly constituted Supreme Court's first bite at an abortion case displayed wanton disregard for the constitutional right to abortion. If anyone had previously been uncertain about what the Court was going to do when it revisited *Roe v. Wade*, the Court showed its hand with the Texas SB8 saga.

OVERTURNING *ROE*

When *Dobbs v. Jackson Women's Health Organization* was argued on December 1, 2022, all eyes were on the Court's newest justices, Brett Kavanaugh and Amy Coney Barrett. There was no doubt that the Court's most liberal members—Justices Breyer, Sotomayor, and Kagan—would vote to strike down the Mississippi law and reaffirm *Roe*. Since Chief Justice Roberts had in 2020 voted to strike down Louisiana's law requiring abortion doctors to have admitting privileges and given his presumed interest in the Court appearing to be a neutral apolitical institution, he was considered a plausible vote to keep *Roe* as well. That meant that at least one of the two newcomers would have to join these four in order for *Roe* to survive.

At oral argument, however, it was hard to see a glimmer of hope in their doing so. Although Chief Justice Roberts floated his idea of a compromise—to uphold the Mississippi ban but keep *Roe*—neither Justice Kavanaugh nor Justice Barrett seemed interested. Instead, Kavanaugh focused on the importance of the Supreme Court remaining neutral in issues of great political controversy, and Barrett posited that laws that allow women to drop newborns at police stations and fire houses to relinquish custody without legal repercussions made abortion no longer necessary.

Five months after argument, a shocking development occurred in the case: *Politico* obtained and published a full draft of the *Dobbs* opinion.[28] The leaked draft indicated it had been written in February by Justice Alito with four other justices joining it—Justices Thomas, Gorsuch, Kavanaugh, and Barrett. The public was stunned, as nothing like this had ever happened before. A leak of *information* about an abortion case was not unprecedented—the *Roe* outcome had been leaked to a *Newsweek* reporter the week before the decision came down, and the outlet accidentally ran the story about the decision a couple of hours before it was announced.[29] However, to leak an entire draft opinion before the final decision was indeed a first.

But the substance of the leaked draft was not much of a shock. Justice Alito's draft opinion explicitly overturned *Roe* and *Casey* and ended constitutional protection for the right to abortion. Theories abounded about the source of the leak. Was it a liberal justice or Court employee looking to spark backlash against the Court hoping to spur one of the Court's conservatives to change their vote? Or was it a conservative justice or Court employee hoping that by releasing the opinion and vote early, it would lock in any possibly wavering members of the majority, who wouldn't want it known that they changed their vote? To this day we don't know the answer because the leaker has not been found.

What we do know is that virtually nothing changed between the leaked opinion and the final version. A month and a half after the leak, on June 24, the Court released its official opinion in *Dobbs*, and the outcome and lineup was the same as in the draft. The Court voted 5–4 to overturn *Roe* and *Casey*, with Justice Alito writing the opinion for himself, Justice Thomas, and the three new Trump appointees, Justices Gorsuch, Kavanaugh, and Barrett. Chief Justice Roberts wrote a concurring opinion that mirrored his position at oral argument. He believed the Mississippi fifteen-week ban was constitutional but that the Court should not take the extra step of overturning *Roe*. Justices Breyer, Sotomayor, and Kagan wrote a joint dissent, arguing that the Mississippi law was unconstitutional and that *Roe* should remain good law.

What did the Court majority say in ultimately overturning *Roe*? Basically, the majority opinion said that it thought *Roe* was "egregiously wrong" and needed to be overturned.[30] The majority found no basis for a right to abortion or privacy in the text of the Constitution. The opinion recognized that in some circumstances courts will interpret broad language from the Constitution to cover rights that are not specifically mentioned, but the majority said that it will only do so when those rights are supported by a historical analysis that shows that history and tradition have protected those rights in the past. Looking back over the centuries, Justice Alito's majority opinion argued that, contrary to Justice Blackmun's historical review in *Roe* and several briefs submitted to the Court on behalf of professional historians, there was a longstanding history of criminalizing abortion both in English common law and in the first century of United States history. In this way, Justice Alito's opinion was the product of the decades-long push by conservative judges and scholars to cement their view of originalism as the only correct way to interpret the Constitution.

Most people believe that the Supreme Court doesn't just overrule a prior case because it's wrong but that it needs a special justification for doing so. Otherwise, law would change too frequently and would appear to be subject to the whims of individual justices. This principle, known as *stare decisis* (literally, "to stand by things decided"), played a major role in *Dobbs* and was the basis for Chief Justice Roberts's separate opinion. But the majority cast precedent aside, primarily because of just how wrong it believed *Roe* to be. Beyond that, the majority claimed that *Roe* and *Casey* in particular had made abortion jurisprudence unworkable. Lower court judges could not discern what was an "undue burden" or "substantial obstacle" without infusing the analysis with their own views. With an incorrect decision that was unworkable, the Court concluded there was no reason to keep *Roe* and *Casey* merely because they were precedent.

With *Roe* and *Casey* overruled, the Court announced the new standard for analyzing restrictions or bans on abortion. Like any claimed right that is not protected by the Constitution, abortion laws would now be analyzed under the "rational basis" test, which allows states and the federal government to enact an abortion restriction or ban abortion as long as there is a legitimate government interest in doing so and the law is rationally related to that interest. This test is the most forgiving test in constitutional law, and almost every law survives it. The majority applied this test to Mississippi's fifteen-week ban and found that it easily passed. According to the majority, the state had an interest in protecting "unborn children," and a ban after fifteen weeks accomplished some of that goal. That suffices under this test, so the law was constitutional.

The joint dissent was furious. The three justices accused the majority of overruling *Roe* not for any legal reasons but rather because of numbers and power. They were unusually sharp in this regard, stating that the "Court reverses course today for one reason and one reason only: because the composition of this Court has changed."[31]

On the legal analysis, the dissent chided the majority for looking for guidance to a historical period when legislatures did not include women and women could not vote. The joint dissent skewered originalism's focus on the time period of the ratification of the Fourteenth Amendment: "But, of course, 'people' did not ratify the Fourteenth Amendment. Men did." They also accused the majority of ignoring the real-world impact this decision would have on women seeking abortions and the chaos that would result from states now having differing laws about abortion.[32]

The varying opinions also battled over the broader impact of overturning *Roe*. Many other rights are protected under the Constitution under the same reasoning as the right to abortion. The right to parent, procreate, make your own medical decisions, sexual intimacy, interracial marriage, same-sex marriage, and more are all rights that the Court has protected despite the absence of explicit guarantees in the Constitution. Justice Alito's majority opinion assured the public that overturning *Roe* would not affect those decisions because, he claimed, abortion is different due to the presence of the fetus.

Justice Thomas, who joined the majority opinion in full, also wrote a separate opinion that no other justice joined explaining his view that almost all of those other rights should be jettisoned along with the right to abortion. To him, they are not grounded in the Constitution's text or history, so they are just as lawless, and the Court "should reconsider all of [its] substantive due process precedents."[33] The joint dissent, expressing concern that Justice Thomas was correct in his view of the implications of the majority opinion for other accepted rights, warned that basic rights taken for granted as an essential part of being a free people were now "under threat."[34]

With *Dobbs*, the almost fifty-year effort to overturn *Roe* accomplished its goal. Through a focused push to appoint antiabortion justices while promoting originalism as a way to combat judicial activism, the antiabortion movement in conjunction with the conservative legal movement finally killed its white whale. But, as the rest of this book shows, although the movement succeeded in ending *Roe*, it has not accomplished its ultimate goal of ending abortion in the United States.

CHAPTER TWO

CLINIC CLOSURES

*And the utter, just ridiculous, absurdity is my
turning into a class A felon overnight if I do
what I spent ten years of training to do.*

—LEAH TORRES, West Alabama
Women's Center

T he most obvious impact of *Dobbs* has been that abortion is now
banned in over a dozen states, and several other states have severely
limited abortion. The impact was swift. The Guttmacher Institute reported that one hundred days after *Dobbs*, over sixty-six clinics in the
states where abortion was now banned had closed or ended their abortion
services.[1] Of those sixty-six clinics, forty were still offering other services
and twenty-six had shut down entirely. The impact these clinic closures
have had and will continue to have on their patients, staff, and communities is immeasurable.

On the one-year anniversary of *Dobbs*, the *New York Times* published a
graphic showing all the clinics that had closed in the past year.[2] It showed
the buildings in small ovals and told the stories of some of the people who
had been employees or patients at the clinics. The collection of all of those
buildings that had been closed or transformed because of *Dobbs*—buildings where people used to provide and receive life-changing care—drove
home exactly what this decision has meant in some parts of the country.

Each and every clinic that stopped providing abortion services in the
wake of *Dobbs*, particularly facilities that offered only abortion services,
employed staff whose lives have been upended by the decision. Like the
patients whose lives have been disrupted because they can no longer get

the care they need in their home states, clinic staff members have had their lives disrupted as well: they've had to close their businesses, stop providing care they are trained to provide, find new jobs, move to a new state, take out loans to survive, and more.

The stories of Andrea Ferrigno and Leah Torres touch on many of these common experiences. And they represent the two main options clinics had in states where abortion bans took effect: shutting the clinic entirely or keeping the doors open but offering different services. Even though their clinics took these different paths, their stories reveal the same ultimate effect: the human cost of being forced to stop providing care to patients, care they would have been able to provide just weeks before. Jody Steinauer's story, which ends this chapter, shows the impact clinic closures because of *Dobbs* have had on training new abortion providers, a loss that may reverberate for a long time into the future.

SHUTTING DOORS

At the moment *Dobbs* was announced, Andrea Ferrigno was riding in a car with her husband and children. Andrea, the vice president of Whole Woman's Health, a network of abortion clinics that started in Texas but had expanded to several more states, had assumed the decision would not be handed down until the following week. When she happened to glance at her phone and saw the news, she had an instantaneous and powerful reaction. "I had to tell my husband to pull over because I had to throw up."

Andrea was thinking in particular about the network's Texas clinics because that's where she herself is based. Andrea's shock was made even more difficult because the Texas ban went into effect so abruptly. "We thought we would have had more time, but the attorney general confirmed that the pre-*Roe* law would go into effect immediately. We tried to challenge that, but the whole challenge lasted a week and then it was done."

Andrea's reaction was so deep because she has spent her entire adult life in abortion care. She came to the United States from Venezuela as a teenager and moved in with her aunt and uncle in McAllen, Texas, a city near the Mexican border. Her uncle was a physician who ran an abortion clinic, and Andrea helped out in the clinic while attending school. After completing her education, she continued to work in the clinic, which was eventually purchased by Whole Woman's Health. Andrea worked in many different capacities as part of Whole Woman's Health, eventually rising to the ranks of corporate vice president.

Whole Woman's Health is an important institution in the history of abortion law in the United States. The organization was the lead plaintiff in two pre-*Dobbs* Supreme Court cases dealing with abortion, *Whole Woman's Health v. Hellerstedt*, a 2016 case that overturned Texas's ambulatory surgical center and admitting privileges law, and *Whole Woman's Health v. Jackson*, the 2021 case that refused to put SB8 on hold.[3] At the time of our first interview with Andrea in early 2022, Whole Woman's Health had brick-and-mortar clinics in Texas, Virginia, Maryland, Minnesota, and Indiana and provided telehealth services in Illinois and New Mexico. Because of *Dobbs*, the Texas clinics were forced to close, and the Indiana clinics became threatened (and ultimately closed a year later, when Indiana's abortion ban went into effect).

Closing the Texas clinics was painful for Andrea, but unfortunately it was not a new experience. When we first spoke to Andrea she was still reeling from years of the Texas legislature's relentless attacks on abortion. "It's been an ongoing thing. It's been draining and exhausting," she said, sighing as she recounted the past fifteen years of the state's abortion wars.

The battles that led to the two Supreme Court cases were especially bruising. The first case, *Whole Woman's Health v. Hellerstedt*, addressed a law that threatened to close nearly all of the forty abortion clinics in the state (not all of them part of the Whole Woman's Health network). The 2013 law required Texas abortion clinics to make hugely expensive upgrades in order to be certified as "ambulatory surgical centers" and also required that all physicians who provided abortions obtain admitting privileges at local hospitals.[4]

The law caused half of the clinics in Texas to shut down immediately and would have had even broader impact had the Supreme Court allowed it to take full effect. Eventually, in 2016, the Supreme Court ruled in Whole Woman's Health's favor, but after the ruling, many of the clinics that had closed were unable to reopen because of staff dispersal and the need to be relicensed. Andrea's clinics struggled to reopen because of these issues and took a long time to get back to normal operations.

But it was a more recent measure, SB8, that was continuing to give her and other Texas abortion providers massive headaches in 2022. It was also, in retrospect, a dress rehearsal for what happened post-*Dobbs*.

SB8 banned abortions after six weeks' gestation, a time during the pregnancy timeline when many women do not know they are pregnant. The most explosive feature of the measure was its enforcement clause, which, rather than putting the law's enforcement in the hands of state and local prosecutors, allowed civil lawsuits instead: *anyone*, anywhere in the world and without any connection to the abortion, could sue a person who performed or aided in the performance of an abortion in violation of the law. The law specifically stated that lawsuits could ask for $10,000 or more as damages.

The draconian nature of SB8, with its threat of almost endless lawsuits and possibly huge fines, inevitably had an impact on the staff of the still-remaining Whole Woman's Health clinics in Texas. Andrea explained to us that there was a lot of confusion among her staff about what constituted aiding an abortion in violation of the law. For example, was it a violation of SB8 to tell a patient over the six-week limit where she might go out of state to get an abortion? As Andrea said, "Even before the law went into effect, we started having trouble with staffing. People were feeling very insecure about what's going to happen. People were thinking about finding other work even outside the field: 'We can't continue to work in abortion care in Texas because it's not reliable.' So we had concerns about retaining staff."

Andrea noted that SB8 led to interesting generational differences among the staff. "We had some staff that have been here for many, many years and went through [the 2013 law] and all of that. They were kind of like, 'Nope, until the last minute, I'm not going anywhere.' But then we have other staff that are younger, that are just now entering the field of reproductive health and abortion care, and this stuff is newish to them. There was a real fear there as to 'What are the implications? How is this going to affect me, my family, and my future?'"

As Andrea made clear to us, it was not just fear of liability that was demoralizing her staff; it was how they were going to have to interact with patients now and deliver to them the terrible news that they couldn't care for them. "Our staff feels terrible," she said. "You have to tell this patient that they can't have an abortion. And you get tired of saying no. And then just at least once a day you want to be able to say 'Yes, let me send you somewhere.'" She summed it up: "When you're the enforcer of a horrible law that you hate, it's just draining."

Not only staff members were unclear about the implications of SB8. Management, including Andrea, was confused as well. She told us they were "trying to understand the implications. How worried should your staff be? How worried should we be? Because this has been such a learning

process, for everybody. Like the attorneys, and the allies, we all were trying to figure out how does it really impact us? To what degree does it
affect us? What happens if we get sued?"

Andrea and other senior staff relied heavily on their attorneys to help
them through this confusing and frightening situation. Attorneys determined that patients who called or came to Whole Woman's Health clinics
in Texas could be referred to the organization's clinics outside the state.
Andrea told us of the network's own "concierge" service that both referred to clinics out of state and helped with patient funding. Andrea and
her colleagues found navigating this landscape very challenging. She acknowledged, with great compassion, the special problems facing immi-
grants who could not so readily leave the state, given the difficulties they
perceived they would face while traveling.

Yet another headache for Andrea was figuring out how to schedule
the doctors who worked at Whole Woman's Health's Texas clinics, nearly
all of whom flew in from out of state. The organization's practice was to
schedule doctors three months in advance. Given that *Dobbs* was only a
few months away and that only six-week abortions were permitted, planning the next round of doctors' schedules was vexing, to say the least.
Andrea worried at the time whether her doctors were going to want to
remain on the schedule. As she explained, "With the [number of proce-
dures] so low, maybe it's not worth it for you to make the trip."

When we ended our conversation with Andrea in early 2022 about the
challenges posed by SB8, one of us jokingly said, "If you think this was a
tough conversation, wait until we talk to you right after *Dobbs*." Andrea
laughed and admitted that her planning around SB8 was in some respects
harder than what would happen if *Roe* was overturned because in early
2022 there was so much uncertainty as to what lay ahead. Whereas if *Roe*
was overturned that year, she said half jokingly, "Should I make a plan for
everything going to hell?"

When *Dobbs* hit, the hell she had worried about was now before her,
and it was harder than she had imagined. After her nausea attack the moment she heard how the case had been decided, the next days involved
more painful episodes.

Perhaps the most personally difficult episode for Andrea was having to
close her beloved McAllen clinic, the facility originally owned by her uncle
where she had begun her own career in abortion care twenty-plus years
earlier. She told us how heartbreaking it was to go to the clinic and hang up

a sign that said "It's been our honor to serve you." As Andrea emotionally described the experience, "It was our goodbye to the community."

Adding to the bitterness of the moment, putting up this new sign involved taking down a sign that Andrea had defiantly posted numerous times over the years in response to Texas's previous attempts to stop abortion: "This clinic stays open. Abortion is still legal." Andrea recounted posting the sign in the past and what a different mindset she had then. "For the last ten years, I can count the number of banners we've had to make where we emphasize this clinic stays open, we're not closing, we're fighting," she told us. "No matter how hard the battle, we always won. So, this time was very different. I've always been able to rely on thinking 'I know it's truly bad right now, but it's going to get better. Like we're going to come out of this. We're going to win. We just have to push through. It'll be fine.'" But now, she said, "We don't have that anymore. There's no light at the end of the tunnel."

Andrea's coping strategy in the aftermath of *Dobbs* was to keep as busy as possible. "I'm just focusing on tactical things, operational things, what do we need to do, who do we need to talk to, what clinic do we pack up, what's the timeline?" One of the most painful tasks she had to do was lay off staff in the various Whole Woman's Health clinics. She was able to keep the McAllen staff employed—many of them had worked there ten years or longer—but in different capacities than their former positions. They shifted to answering phones for the organization's call center, helping with the organization's Abortion Wayfinder Program, which offered various kinds of practical assistance, and doing some advocacy work. Though gratified that she could keep some staff on the payroll, Andrea admitted these new positions were not ideal for veteran staff. "It is not what they signed up to do. They didn't apply for a call center job when they started working on abortion. They wanted that one-on-one interaction with the patient. It's what they've always done."

Later in 2022, Andrea faced one of her most difficult post-*Dobbs* situations with this particular clinic. Once the McAllen clinic closed, Whole Woman's Health eventually decided that it was best for the organization to sell that property. Andrea explained that there had been particular pressure to sell the McAllen building quickly. The staff had been working in the building answering calls, but Andrea grew concerned about continued state harassment. "The state showed up to make sure we weren't doing any abortions," she told us. "We told them no, and they were like, 'Well, why are you here?' and it just made us nervous and we realized we can't be here. So we moved everyone to remote." She also explained that selling the clinic was necessary to keep the McAllen employees on the payroll. Andrea commiserated with staff saying good-bye to the physical clinic. "That's your second home. You spend more time at the clinic than you spend in your house, and now you have to pack it all up."

Simply selling the property was incredibly challenging for Andrea: this was her beloved McAllen clinic, the clinic that was so embedded in her family history. This painful situation became considerably worse when the group that bought the clinic—who Andrea and others at Whole Woman's Health had been led to believe would open a family medicine practice serving the local community—turned around and, within a few weeks of purchasing the property, sold the building to a crisis pregnancy center that planned to operate a fake clinic there.

Andrea was devastated. She had initially been comforted by the belief that people could still go to that location for medical care, even if not abortion care. But now that an antiabortion fake clinic was going to operate out of the site, Andrea's sorrow from such a tough year ran even deeper. After this sale, Andrea was unable to visit McAllen for over a year, and when she eventually did visit family there, she steered clear of downtown to avoid the painful memory.

When we asked Andrea if it was feasible to turn the Texas abortion clinics in the Whole Woman's Health organization into a general obstetrics and gynecology or other sexual health facility, she explained to us that the organization had tried such a conversion previously and it didn't go well. After the 2013 Texas law that resulted in the closure of many clinics throughout the state, Whole Woman's Health tried to keep the McAllen clinic open for non-abortion care, but it was only financially sustainable for three months. "You can't pay the bills doing Pap smears," Andrea said.

But what about the patients? Andrea and her colleagues immediately had to figure out what they were allowed to say to Texas patients who called seeking an abortion appointment. The call center and Wayfinder program receive calls from people all over the country. While dealing with callers from other states was straightforward, dealing with Texans was more complicated. After much discussion with lawyers—discussions that had begun earlier because of SB8—Andrea told us that Whole Woman's Health staff could legally provide information to Texans as well as others, but that this understanding could change.

As Andrea admitted, "We're constantly going back to our attorneys to see if that's all right." She was always on the lookout for antiabortion "plants" who would call Whole Woman's Health and try to entrap a staff member into saying something that could be construed as illegal, but she wasn't too worried about this. As she wryly explained, "They can't even play patient right! They'll ask if we are going to do an ultrasound to confirm there is no heartbeat? Patients never ask that!"

By the end of 2022, Andrea and her team had figured out how to use technology to solve some of these issues. Texas's various overlapping abortion bans imposed delicate maneuvering on the call centers, but the new technology the call centers employed identified the state in which the caller was located, so staff could route callers to an operator on the basis of what the caller was asking for. "So I could be in Texas and I could give somebody information where they could go. That's not a problem. But when it comes to scheduling, funding, consenting, there are some limitations there. And so we would transfer that call to a staff person in a safe state."

Because of the close work Andrea does with the people who staff the call centers, she had a great vantage point for observing patient patterns in the face of clinic closures. For Whole Woman's Health patients who have been forced to travel because of the Texas closures, Andrea noted what others in the post-*Dobbs* era have also reported: where feasible, patients in states where abortion is banned prefer driving to get an abortion in a state where it remains legal, rather than flying. In part this is because patients are often traveling with family. "When your childcare is also the person that needs to go with you because you need an escort [as patients typically do for second-trimester procedures], . . . the whole family gets in the car and they go. And the patient goes in to have the abortion, and the family is in the car waiting." She also mentioned that, for Texans driving is a way of life, whereas dealing with flying, especially airport security, can be overwhelming for some.

To those for whom the choice of transportation did not matter, Andrea explained that the prime issue was getting an abortion as fast as possible. Referring to how patients have been thinking about the issue, Andrea said, "If I can have an appointment in Virginia on Tuesday, but get one in California on Monday, I'm going to go [to California]. Because I just want the fastest appointment I can."

As 2022 progressed, Andrea and others at Whole Woman's Health attempted to open a new clinic in a small town in New Mexico, just over the Texas border, to help support the Texas patients. In this effort Whole Woman's Health faced what a number of other abortion providers looking to relocate did—a concerted campaign by antiabortion organizers to mobilize local opposition to establishing clinics in border towns, which are often rural and conservative.

Whole Woman's Health was in the process of acquiring a building and applying for a clinic license when local pro-choice activists raised concerns about the wisdom of such a move for the local community, given the fierce opposition. "They were very concerned about safety and the fact that we might not get any support from local authorities, who might be part of what puts us in danger." Whole Woman's Health pulled out of the planned move and instead decided to open a clinic in Albuquerque, where a number of other providers from states with bans had already relocated. Albuquerque was a much more supportive environment, but Andrea regretted how much farther Texas residents would have to drive to get there.

The toll that these battles had taken on Whole Woman's Health's workforce as a whole was something that Andrea kept returning to when we talked with her. She voiced her concern and sympathy for the abortion-providing workforce, not just in Texas, where clinics had closed, but also in states where abortion remained legal. She noted that the provider community had already gone through the upheaval of the pandemic: "They worked straight through, never took a break. And now *Roe* falling and [they're] going through another trauma?"

She noted that a number of her organization's doctors were experiencing burnout and had requested a leave of absence, which she was happy to grant. And she wondered how reentry was going to be for them, given the huge caseloads at some clinics in states that would be absorbing all the travelers. The providers were "making all these crazy trips from one end of the world to the next." As she put it, "There's only so much time you can spend at the beach. Then you come back home and back to reality, and how is that going to be? Once you've had time to settle down and realize all the shit you just went through?" Then, laughing, she returned to her own survival strategy. "That's why I don't stop. Because if I stop to think about it, I don't know that I'll be able to get up again. So, I just don't."

CHANGING CARE MODEL

For Andrea and her colleagues, closing their Texas clinics and trying to find their staff other positions within the organization was the best response to

Dobbs for their situation. According to the *New York Times*, one year after *Dobbs* about half of the clinics in states with abortion bans had taken this approach.[5] But, importantly, not all chose to close. Others moved to a more hospitable location, something that we will cover in the next chapter.

But others tried something else: continuing to operate but without providing abortion care. Leah Torres told us this is the approach West Alabama Women's Center has taken in the wake of *Dobbs*. Leah is a doctor who serves as the medical director of the clinic, a position she held before *Dobbs*. Leah's story of what happened because of *Dobbs* shows the challenges clinics face transitioning to another slate of care. It also shows the human costs of being forced to give up your life's work.

Leah heard the news about *Roe* being overturned when she was already in a very difficult place. On that day she was in transit, returning to Alabama after a visit to her family. The unplanned visit was a sad one, as a family member had died. While stopping off at a relative's house on her way back home, she happened to glance at her phone and saw the news. "In a wave, it hit me: you are not a citizen, equal under the law. And my profession became a criminal act."

When we asked how she was now processing *Dobbs* when we spoke to her several weeks later, she replied, "You might as well ask me, 'How do you process the fact that aliens have landed on our planet?'" Making matters even more emotionally difficult, shortly after the decision Leah received a death threat on a social media platform. She immediately reported this threat to the National Abortion Federation, who contacted the FBI.

Leah had been working at West Alabama Women's Center only since 2020, but her tenure had already been tumultuous. Leah had known from an early age that she was going to be a medical-care professional; a women's studies course in college and involvement with the organization Medical Students for Choice in medical school put her on the path of becoming an abortion provider. After training as an obstetrician-gynecologist, she took a fellowship in family planning in Utah.

"I'm really glad I trained in Utah and not, for example, in California," she said. "I thought, 'What insanity is this? I'm going to Salt Lake City to learn how to do abortions?' However, it gave me very important skills." She expressed gratitude for learning how to navigate Utah's hostile-to-abortion politicians, community members, and hospital executives.

But she didn't stay in Utah forever. She needed to move after a tweet of hers about later (post–first trimester) abortions went viral and attracted too much antiabortion attention to her employer. She moved to New Mexico, where she did not perform abortions but earned some money toward paying off her medical school debt. When the job in Alabama opened in early 2020, she jumped at the opportunity. "Alabama comes along," she explained, "and says, 'Hey, do you want this dream job?' So of course I said, 'Bye, New Mexico, see you later.' Because this was the first opportunity that I had to incorporate abortion into my general care. And I was going to be calling the shots. You mean, I can just do things because it's evidence based? I don't have to get permission from multiple administrators who don't know what they're talking about? Sign me up."

Unfortunately for Leah, it wasn't so easy going when she got to Alabama. From the moment she got there, she encountered resistance from state officials, a resistance she attributed to abortion politics. Her temporary license to practice was revoked, and her application for a permanent license was denied—health department officials claimed she had committed "fraud" in filling out the necessary paperwork. Only after about a year of hassles from state bureaucrats—and over $100,000 in lawyer's fees—did she get her license, along with a written acknowledgment that her license should never have been held up in the first place.

Unsurprisingly, this experience left her outraged at how Alabama's abortion politics impact care for everyone, especially the Black and impoverished patients who came to her clinic. Reflecting on the struggle over her license, she said, "This is August 2020, in the middle of a pandemic, and they've got everybody calling for volunteers, for physicians and nurses to volunteer to give out vaccine shots. And I'm extremely frustrated thinking, well, had you not taken my license, I could've helped, but, you know, apparently, you don't need my help."

She also has been profoundly affected by the deep racism in healthcare in her new home state. "Working in Alabama has been a huge learning experience. The racism is frightening. It's palpable, and it's just horrifying to see it in action. I've seen already why Alabama is number three in the maternal mortality rate." And yet, Leah explained, the state is so focused on stopping abortion that it doesn't focus on any other health issues. "Healthcare here is bad, and they're all focused on making abortion go away, and yet Alabama has one of the highest heart attack rates, and rates for chronic health conditions."

Leah also struggled upon arriving in Alabama with her relationship with other medical establishments. She sought a closer relationship between her

freestanding abortion clinic and a local hospital so that she could more easily refer challenging cases to them, but this was not in the cards. Like other
abortion providers around the country, she was unable to obtain privileges
at any nearby hospital. She simultaneously tried fruitlessly to establish a
relationship with the county health department, and only after a nearly
yearlong effort was she able to get Medicaid approval for her non-abortion
services. She attributed all these obstacles to the fact that she was a doctor
in a facility that mainly provided abortions.

Given the extreme social problems that seemingly affected many of her
clinic's patients, this isolation from other medical institutions was a real
problem. This was especially true of some of the youngest patients Leah
saw, who were victims of rape and incest. Leah's policy was to use only local
sedation in her clinic, but she felt that these youngest patients would benefit
from a higher degree of sedation. When she was faced with a young teen
who had been raped by her mother's boyfriend, she felt that "a thirteen-
year-old should not be awake in any way, shape, or form for this procedure." She knew that sending this patient to the nearest hospital was not
an option because the obstetrics and gynecology department chair at that
hospital was also the medical director of the local antiabortion fake clinic.

Appealing to a university-affiliated hospital an hour or so away also
proved useless. While she was in the process of negotiating with the maternal fetal division head about the thirteen-year-old's care, the next day
a fifteen-year-old who had been raped by her brother came to her clinic.
Leah frantically again emailed the division head at the university hospital.
She paraphrased the email for us: "I'm sorry for the follow-up so quickly,
but I have another young patient, so I need for you to get back to me
quickly on how we can collaborate to help Alabamians. What is your
hospital's policy? I am a community provider and I need to know what
resources there are and where to send patients."

The doctor in question finally called and said his hospital would not
accept either patient, telling her, "It's not a legal issue. It's because the
staff won't do it, and I can't make them." Leah ultimately found another
provider, several hours away, who agreed to care for the thirteen-year-old
with the higher degree of sedation that Leah sought for the patient. But
Leah reluctantly performed the abortion on the older teen herself, wish-
ing she could offer more sedation. "I don't want to re-traumatize these
patients. They don't need to be awake, with the speculum inserted and a
stranger in their vagina." At the same time, she explained, "I don't want

to use IV sedation because the state has made me very afraid of taking on any more risk."

Even before *Dobbs* Leah was already familiar with the impact abortion bans and a hostile environment had on her patients. Her clinic was very busy in the months leading up to *Dobbs* because of the many patients arriving from Texas where abortion after six weeks was unavailable due to SB8. Moreover, clinic staff constantly dealt with aggressive protesters, and they had to respond to the ongoing attempts of the Alabama legislature to further regulate abortion.

So when the Supreme Court overturned *Roe*, Leah was already very familiar with the challenges of being a provider in a hostile environment. But this time even bigger hurdles were before her. Once she returned to the clinic after her visit with her family, Leah had to work through figuring out with coworkers and an attorney what now constituted care that the clinic could legally offer, comforting the distraught staff, as well as managing her own emotions and confronting the long-term prospects for the clinic. Alabama had a "trigger law" whereby abortion would become illegal in the state as soon as *Roe* was overturned. So new protocols had to be put in place immediately.

Leah was acutely aware of the stakes involved if she were to be found guilty of performing an abortion that would be considered illegal in Alabama: she could be sentenced to up to ninety-nine years in prison. She also was cognizant of the fact that the attorney general had announced, as she paraphrased it, "Any state attorneys that are not going to prosecute abortion providers will get prosecuted themselves."

We asked her about the one exception for an abortion that her state now allowed, a threat to a pregnant woman's life, and what that concretely meant. She answered, "I don't know what that means. The attorney general doesn't know what it means, but it doesn't matter. Because it's going to mean whatever they want it to mean, in whatever scenario they want it to mean it in." She speculated that there would likely be selective prosecution for such abortions that did take place. Referring to her earlier struggle over her license when she first arrived in the state, she predicted that if doctors who were known to be antiabortion actually did perform an abortion to save a life, they would not be prosecuted. "I do the same procedure and I'm in cuffs, being thrown in jail."

Leah's clear-eyed recognition of her inability to continue to provide abortions in Alabama led her to ruminate with us about alternative life planning. She told us she had renewed her license in a state where abortion remained legal. She also, to our surprise, raised the possibility of leaving medicine altogether, making clear her disillusionment with the current healthcare system in ways that go well beyond bans on abortion. Reflecting on what her time in Alabama has conveyed to her, she said, "What I'm hearing is that helping people doesn't matter, and helping people is why I went into medicine." Unfortunately, she explained, "that's not what healthcare in this country is about. We're about making hospitals profitable. We're about paying pharmaceutical companies. And we want insurance companies to profit. And doctors have no say in anything, patients even less." She raised the possibility of becoming a national park ranger or perhaps writing a book about the healthcare system, in particular the field of obstetrics and gynecology and its treatment of patients.

As of the end of 2022, though, Leah was sticking with her clinic in Alabama. "This is where I live until I can't afford it anymore, because I am out of a job." A major reason for this commitment is the deep bond that exists among Leah and the other staff members of West Alabama Women's Center. "When you are in this work, you're family," she said. "When you're in this work in the South and you're under fire on a day-to-day basis, you know, you become really close to the people you work with."

But sticking with it required changing how the clinic operated, because now it couldn't provide abortions. Making these changes was what she and her colleagues spent their time doing in the aftermath of *Dobbs*. Leah reminded us that the intent behind her initial hiring by this clinic in 2020 was to expand the facility's services beyond abortion. So early in her arrival in Alabama, while she was waiting for the resolution of her license dispute, she expanded her training in a number of areas, including HIV care and gender-affirming care for trans patients. She told us that through a combination of successful fundraising and careful budgeting in anticipation of the overturning of *Roe*, the clinic actually had the resources to remain open for at least a short period of time after the cessation of abortion care.

The major challenge with staying open after *Dobbs*, Leah explained, involved a serious "rebranding" of the clinic. "For thirty years, everyone has known us as an abortion clinic," and now the task was to get out the word about the other services provided, and to be explicit that the clinic did not provide abortions. A major stumbling block for this expansion of services was a bureaucratic entanglement with Medicaid. As Leah explained the Kafkaesque situation, Medicaid of Alabama had *approved* her as a Medicaid provider in December 2020, but when we spoke in July 2022, just after *Dobbs*, they still had not *enrolled* her. She told us of a number of frustrating delays—"I don't know how many times we've redone the enrollment form"—which she attributed to antiabortion politics. Because she was the only physician, Leah's not having full status as a Medicaid enrollee meant that the clinic would receive no financial reimbursement for providing the necessary healthcare to Alabama's largely impoverished patients for the array of non-abortion services the clinic now offered.

The problem with Medicaid was finally resolved by the end of 2022. This came about after another bruising legal battle, Leah told us. The clinic, no longer an abortion-providing establishment, was able to forge relationships with other major insurers besides Medicaid. At the end of 2022 the clinic was trying to survive as a multiservice gynecological clinic that did nearly everything in that field—except abortions. Leah noted one positive result of the post-*Dobbs* rebranding: the clinic no longer had to deal with protesters, although the antiabortion fake clinic next door *still* tried to lure unsuspecting patients to enter its doors.

Leah rattled off the services the clinic now provided: all forms of birth control, prenatal care (though not deliveries), Pap smear screenings and colposcopy, sexually transmitted infection screening, trans healthcare, gender-affirming care, telehealth appointments, HIV care, and prescribing PrEP (pre-exposure prophylaxis to prevent HIV). She told us she was committed to developing new skills. "I am definitely trying to do things that my patients are asking for." She told of learning to inject Botox and filler for trans patients as well as hormone pellet insertion, a new technique Leah learned in response to a patient request.

Financial viability was a huge issue for the clinic. She said that having ties with various insurance providers was very useful but admitted, "I'm not seeing as many patients as I want to see. So I'm expanding my skills because I can and because we need whatever revenue we can get." Leah was concerned that there were not more funds available for advertising, which was needed to get more patients through the door. At the end of 2022, Leah said, the clinic had raised enough funding to stay open through June 2023, but she wasn't sure at that time if the clinic could remain open beyond that date. (As of June 2024 the clinic was still open and operating, and still fundraising to stay that way.)

Like many of the people we interviewed for this book, Leah was very concerned about clinic staff and their employment possibilities if the clinic were to eventually close. She was gratified they were still employed, even after *Dobbs*, and, importantly, were learning new skills that could help with future employment if necessary. As she said, "They're not doing what they signed up for"—acknowledging that the staff was deeply committed to, and missed, abortion work. But she pointed to a medical assistant who had recently completed a course that permitted her to do blood draws. Reflecting on the staff's dedication to its new mission of "any and all needed healthcare," Leah told us, "I'm so proud of our clinic and what we have always stood for: unfettered access to healthcare."

Despite her pride in the clinic's new mission, Leah was still confused about how the clinic should deal with abortion in this post-*Dobbs* reality and angry about the patients they could no longer adequately serve. Obviously, the clinic no longer offered abortions (which it still states prominently on its website: "WAWC does NOT provide elective abortions"). But the issue of abortion referrals after *Dobbs* was confusing. The clinic's attorney's recommendation was that patients who had completed the first visit for an abortion pre-*Dobbs* (Alabama required two) could be given a referral, under the principle of "continuity of care."

Although the lawyer advised that anyone already scheduled could be referred elsewhere, he cautioned the clinic staff not to give such information to anyone else. This put staff in the difficult position of withholding information they very much wanted to give their patients. As Leah put it, with incredulity, "I can't provide medical information to people?" An added twist was the fear that "antis will call and try to trap us." She reconstructed, with evident frustration, a call she had answered earlier in the day that we spoke right after *Dobbs*: "They asked, 'So, I know that this thing went down. Does that mean that no abortions can happen?' And I have to choose my words carefully and say, 'According to Alabama state law, abortion is illegal in this state.' Of course the next question is, 'So, where can I get information?' and I have to use vague language and present myself as aloof, like, 'I don't know. I mean, you might be able to look online.'" In short, Leah thought that being purposely vague was her best legal strategy, although she bitterly resented having to do so.

After more time had passed, post-*Dobbs*, to Leah there still remained some ambiguity as to whether the staff could refer for abortions. In mid-2023, months after we had last interviewed Leah, her clinic, two others in Alabama, and the state's abortion fund sued the state attorney general over this issue.[6] The state attorney general had threatened to prosecute anyone giving a referral to or aiding someone to get an abortion in another state. The still-pending lawsuit alleges that this threat violates the federal constitutional right to travel and speech.

Both the ambiguity around referrals and Leah's furor at being unable to take care of patients were revealed in an incident she recounted for us:

So I had a patient come in. She was forty-four years old, about to be forty-five, and she's pregnant. And she did everything that she was supposed to. Took the birth control, used condoms, and she's just devastated. Devastated. She has a grown adult child in their twenties. She absolutely does not want to be pregnant. She's crying, and she's upset. I can't describe how it feels to say this, but in my mind, I have to think about "What if she's a plant? She could be a plant. She could be an anti."

But in the end, I am going to be me and I said, "You know what? Ethically, and morally, and—according to medical ethics—it is safer for you to have an abortion [than to complete a pregnancy]. And I should be able to tell you that, and so, I'm telling you that. Because, according to medical ethics, if you want an abortion, that's exactly what I would support you in doing. That is actually safest for you. There are much higher risks of you experiencing a whole bunch of health problems continuing this pregnancy and giving birth. I can't tell you what to do, but for what it's worth, I'm glad you would like an abortion. I'm sorry I can't help you with that, but I'm glad that you would like one."

In my mind, I'm not a lawyer, but I am a fellowship-trained physician who specializes in reproductive health. This is my wheelhouse. So, I said, "The internet has a vast amount of information and resources on it, say, for example, if someone wanted to get abortion pills. One could go to this website, or that website." Generally, I tell people to be careful of their browser. And maybe go to the library and use the computer there. Clear browsing data. Take digital security precautions.

I sent her to our website, which has resources for prenatal care, adoption services, and abortion care. The conversation was awkward, to say the least, and I explained to her, "You could be a plant, and this is something I have to think about, unfortunately. Even so, this is beyond that. Your health and life matter. I'm telling you what you should do in order to procure the care you decide you need, and abortion is illegal in this state for me to provide for you. But you have resources. Here they are."

Reflecting on this incident, Leah told us she felt it was her professional obligation to counsel the patient in that way, saying heatedly, "I'm over it, I'm over putting other people's lives in danger because men have decided they know what pregnancy is about. Every day the government finds more ways to make saving lives a criminal act. Who knew medical school, residency, and fellowship training would lead to prison because of the zip code you practice in?" She acknowledged that she did not consult with the rest of the staff before this conversation with the patient, not wanting them to assume any liability, should there be any follow-up. She also pointed out the irony of having 240 tablets of mifepristone—the first drug in the two-drug regimen used in a medication abortion—in a cabinet at the clinic and being unable to use these pills to help the forty-four-year-old patient with her unwanted pregnancy.

Leah did use one of these mifepristone doses to aid a patient in the midst of a miscarriage, a recognized use of the drug. On the one hand, she knew that what she was doing was appropriate. "I gave her the mifepristone because medically, that's what I am supposed to do. And legally, I didn't break the law." On the other hand, she still had some wariness of how Alabama officials might respond to this, if they somehow found out about her dispensation of mifepristone. If they wanted to prosecute her, she speculated, "they're going to do it anyway. If they decide up is down, north is south, I can't control that. I learned that when I first moved here."

The emotional toll on Leah of no longer being able to properly take care of her patients was devastating. "I couldn't have anticipated what that would be like. I knew it was going to be hard. But when you've got someone who has six kids already, doesn't speak English, can't read or write in her own native language, begging for help with not having a seventh child—nothing can prepare you for what that's like." But she remained steadfast that she wasn't going to abandon Alabama or her patients there. "I'm going to do everything I can to stay here because people here—even outside of abortion—are suffering. They're not getting the healthcare they need. I don't want to leave a void."

Despite her resolution to stay in Alabama as long as it was feasible to keep the clinic afloat, Leah made it very clear that not being able to perform abortions was a real loss for her. To Leah, abortion care "is part of my heart and soul. It is a special calling for me."

ABORTION TRAINING IN CRISIS

Dobbs has had yet another negative effect beyond the immediate impact on pregnant women and providers. Clinics closing or no longer providing abortion care in states with abortion bans has shut off what has historically been one of the main venues for abortion training for obstetrics and gynecology residents in those states.

In the years immediately following *Roe*, despite abortion's being a common procedure, hospitals did not immediately mandate routine abortion training for their residents in obstetrics and gynecology, the specialty most associated with abortion care—a reflection of the conflict-averse nature of that field at the time. Nor did a majority of hospitals establish on-site routine abortion care, only offering such care to the relatively small number of women who were very ill or who were carrying a severely compromised fetus.

Not until 1996, more than twenty years after *Roe*, did the medical associations tasked with setting standards for this field establish a requirement for abortion training, with opt-out possibilities for those with religious or moral objections. But in a stunning example of "abortion exceptionalism"—treating abortion differently from other healthcare services—Congress took the unprecedented step of blunting the force of the new requirement by passing an amendment stipulating that residencies that did not comply would not lose federal funding or accreditation.[7]

In 1999, in response to the uneven level of training in US programs, abortion advocates within obstetrics and gynecology circles established the Kenneth J. Ryan Residency Training Program (named for a trailblazing abortion doctor). The Ryan Program, as it is called, raises private funding to support programs across the country in implementing the training mandate. The program is now present in 38 percent of US obstetrics and gynecology residencies. Over the years it has introduced hundreds of young physicians to abortion care. Since fewer than 5 percent of abortions in the United States take place in hospitals, the Ryan Program and its cooperating residency programs have adapted by integrating stand-alone abortion clinics as sites for training. But the closure of facilities in the wake of *Dobbs* has made such clinic-based training impossible in states that ban abortions.

Jody Steinauer has felt this impact almost personally. Jody is an obstetrics and gynecology professor at the University of California, San Francisco, and the director of the Ryan Program. As a medical student in the

1990s, Jody was one of the founders of Medical Students for Choice and has remained passionate about the need for abortion training.

Anticipating the overturn of *Roe*, Jody was naturally worried both about what would become of the training that had formerly taken place in the states with bans and what would become of those who needed abortion care. In states without abortion clinics, she explained to us when we talked with her two weeks before *Dobbs* was decided, hospitals are going to be critical sites for providing whatever legal abortion care would be permissible, so she feels it essential that residents there receive training in performing abortions wherever possible. She pointed out that about 44 percent of obstetrics and gynecology residents are in states where abortion is likely to be banned. Since medical residents often remain in the states where they trained, she worries that these states will not have clinicians able to take care of the pregnancy-related emergencies that demand knowledge of more complex abortion procedures.

But her concerns about the future of abortion training go beyond abortion itself. As she put it, "The reason that we have to try as hard as we can to make sure those residents learn these skills is obviously for future abortion care, but also for pregnancy-loss care and for pregnancy-related emergencies." Jody told us of interesting recent research with which she was involved that revealed that obstetrics and gynecology residents who had completed routine abortion training felt more confident than those without such training in performing *other* skills in the specialty, particularly miscarriage management.[8] Treating a patient with a miscarriage is similar to performing a first-trimester procedural abortion.

Moreover, mifepristone and misoprostol, the drugs used in medication abortion, have other obstetrical uses, including in the treatment of miscarriages, leading Jody to urge her Ryan Program colleagues to ensure that their hospital pharmacies stock these drugs. She told us that she hoped that hospital residency directors in states with abortion bans understand that if *Roe* was overturned they were "going to see more people with bleeding" from miscarriages as well as from using abortion pills obtained through various means. She hoped that the directors would understand that "you're not going to be able to send your residents to their local clinic to get their abortion training, so let's do better by the patients who are going to need your services and train the residents."

Jody laid out the Ryan Program's two-pronged strategy to deal with the predicted coming crisis in states with bans. The first prong is to help program-affiliated faculty in those states negotiate with numerous other entities in their hospitals to manage the earthquake in obstetrical care that the decision would create. This prong continues to this day. The second is to arrange out-of-state training, to the extent possible, for residents in states with bans.

Neither of these strategies is simple. The first recommendation the program made to its affiliates in states with bans was to develop an institutional task force drawn from many sectors of the academic medical center—president, deans, department chairs, hospital counsel, and so on—to try to develop some consensus on which abortions would be legally permitted even with an abortion ban in place. Despite these efforts, such a consensus has been very hard to achieve. Faculty are also urged to develop referral pathways for patients and to identify in advance states to which they could send patients who did not meet the criteria for an authorized abortion.

The issue of the care of patients who present with problems after using abortion pills on their own has been a particular concern of Jody and her colleagues. Abortion pills are safe and effective and have a very low complication rate; however, patients sometimes present to emergency departments with worries about too much bleeding. Although the physical condition of someone who is having a naturally occurring miscarriage is typically indistinguishable from that of someone who has taken abortion pills, if the latter admit to having taken pills in a state with an abortion ban, there have been instances where emergency department staff reported these patients to the police. Therefore, Jody sees a key mission of Ryan Program faculty to be educating emergency department colleagues not to report such patients: reporting people seeking healthcare to the criminal justice system can reduce people's willingness to seek healthcare in the first place.

The second strategy, sending residents out of state for training, had started before *Dobbs* because of SB8, which made in-state training in Texas virtually impossible. But, Jody acknowledged, arranging out-of-state training can be cumbersome. Ryan Program staff shared with us a four-page single-spaced document that specified the numerous issues that had to be addressed by a residency program in order to send a trainee to a program in a state where abortion is legal, including issues of liability, contract, salary, licensing, personal background checks on the trainee, and more.

Of course, not all residents have the capacity to leave town for a month or longer for training, especially if they have family responsibilities. In all medical fields, training students typically slows down the provision of care, and some programs in states where abortion remains legal, anticipating a huge influx of patients post-*Dobbs*, are hesitant to take on additional residents. Nevertheless, by the end of 2023 around 130 residents from states with bans have been able to obtain training in programs in legal states and the numbers continue to grow. While this number is impressive, given the numerous barriers that must be overcome, it falls far short of the roughly 300 residents a year from states with bans that the Ryan Program would ideally like to see receiving abortion training.

Jody focuses on the crisis in training for obstetricians-gynecologists, but family medicine physicians and advanced practice clinicians—physician assistants, nurse midwives, and nurse practitioners—also play a significant role in abortion provision. Training for these groups has long been less routinized than that for obstetrician-gynecologists, and the closure of clinics after *Dobbs* will make that situation even worse.

DISILLUSIONMENT AND DETERMINATION

Returning to Andrea and Leah, the events of 2022 were deeply disillusioning and disappointing, as they were for their peers elsewhere in the country.[9] They have both dedicated their entire adult lives to the core task of taking care of people who need a medical care provider's help. To describe how she was feeling now that she couldn't offer that help, help she was capable of providing, Leah said it's like "being in a boat, and you see someone in the water who's drowning. And you are about to throw them a life jacket, but somebody is saying, 'You're not allowed to throw the life jacket.'"

The disillusionment Andrea feels now that *Roe* has been overturned is interwoven with her feelings about being an immigrant. Describing the challenges of coming to a new country at a young age without her parents, she said it was nonetheless worth it. "You are making sacrifices for a better life, a better future, a place where human rights are protected and the laws matter." Despite making clear to us that she was very grateful for her US citizenship and that she still loved being a Texan, she was utterly stunned at the betrayal *Dobbs* represented. As she said to us in disbelief, speaking of conservatives both on the Court and in politics, "As crazy as they are, they at least have to respect the Constitution."

Despite the setbacks, both Andrea and Leah made clear that they still have a role to play in reproductive health. Leah will remain with her clinic as long as it is financially feasible but also plans to keep up her skills as an abortion provider, with occasional stints in states where abortion is legal. Andrea continues to play a central role in Whole Woman's Health operations in states where abortion remains legal. Jody had a different twist on the ongoing work, calling herself "optimistic because everyone is just trying so hard, and they are just systematically working on it."

However, their determination and hard work notwithstanding, these committed individuals, like every other person who provided abortions for people in states where it is now banned, are facing a fast-changing and hostile environment. Leah mentioned to us that she obtained a Florida medical license in the hopes of providing abortion care there part-time. But in 2023, Florida passed a law banning abortions after six weeks, and the law went into effect in May 2024.

Likewise, Andrea told us that she and her colleagues were thinking of opening a clinic in North Carolina and had started preliminary investigations of a location. But in 2023, North Carolina passed a twelve-week abortion ban, making the prospect of opening a new clinic that much more difficult. Andrea's and Leah's uncertain futures in their chosen life's work drives home a point Andrea made to us about living through the overturning of *Roe* and having to close abortion clinics in her home state: "You asked me earlier if the situation could get any worse. Yes. More safe states could be gone."

CHAPTER THREE

CREATIVE ALTERNATIVES

*In Wyoming, we are going to litigate, we are going
to fight this thing to the end, and we're going to
see hopefully if we can hold the line there.*

—JULIE BURKHART, Wellspring Health Access

Not every abortion provider in a state with an abortion ban has shut
down or stopped providing abortion services. Some abortion providers operating in states that banned abortion after *Dobbs* have taken advantage of their unique environments to continue their life's work through
creative measures.

These individuals have found various ways to continue to make abortion as accessible as possible for their patients. Their creative responses to
Dobbs are a significant contributor to the increase in abortion numbers after
Roe was overturned. One way that many clinics have survived is by moving
to a state without an abortion ban, an option chosen by clinic directors and
owners in Tennessee, Mississippi, and Texas, to name just a few.

This is not to suggest that such a move is always simple. Some communities in non-restricted states that are located on the border of states with
bans have made it clear that new clinics are not welcome. In the previous
chapter, this is what happened to Andrea Ferrigno when Whole Woman's
Health planned a move to a border town in New Mexico but was thwarted
by local conditions.

But even when there is not significant local resistance, such a move can
be complicated. The three longtime abortion providers featured in this
chapter, all of whom have been active in this field for at least thirty years,

were able to come up with creative solutions and successfully navigate *Dobbs*. Their stories illustrate the importance of allies if creativity in the face of oppression is to succeed.

All three of the providers in this chapter have remained committed to this work, despite varying degrees of harassment and threats by abortion opponents, including, in two cases, having their workplaces firebombed. All responded to the *Dobbs* decision with considerable creativity—in two cases by deftly shifting their operations to states where abortion remains legal, and in the other, by having the fortitude to embark on opening a clinic in a state where the status of legal abortion remains unclear. Their stories reveal these providers' staunch determination to push back against the limitations brought by *Dobbs*. Their stories also show that the full impact of this decision remains very much in flux, subject to local changes and legal rulings still to come. Despite these successes, it is still an open question whether some of these new ventures will succeed.

MOVING ACROSS THE STATE LINE

Tammi Kromenaker will never forget the patient who called just after *Dobbs* was decided. Tammi, the owner and director of the Red River Women's Clinic, was in the clinic's Fargo, North Dakota, office the morning the Supreme Court announced its decision. In the days leading up to the decision, she had been monitoring the Supreme Court's website on a daily basis in her office in anticipation of what the Court might do. When the news came that morning just after 9 a.m. central time, she called the two staff members who were with her that day into her office and shouted to her colleagues, "Oh, my God, you guys, we have *Dobbs*!"

The three of them together at the clinic were "very upset and crying and angry. And then the phone rang. All three lines were going." The other staff members answered the first two calls, so it was up to Tammi to answer the third. "I had to answer the phone within thirty seconds of finding out that *Roe v. Wade* had been overturned. And this person said, 'I need to make an appointment.' And of course, she had no idea [that *Dobbs* had just been decided]. And I started making her appointment, and I was having a really hard time holding it together."

As Tammi struggled to make the appointment, her husband called her on her cell phone. She put the patient on hold and took his call. "I just started bawling to him. And he said, 'We knew this was coming. We've got a plan. We're going to get through this.' So, I took a really big breath, said 'Thank you, that's what I needed to hear,' and I went back and made the patient's appointment." Although Tammi managed to remain composed while making the appointment, immediately afterwards the news really hit. She gathered again with the two in-office staff, and "we hugged and cried and swore."

The patient Tammi scheduled that morning continued to have symbolic importance to her as an affirmation that people will still need abortions and that such care will continue to be provided. When this patient came in the following week for her abortion—North Dakota's ban had not yet kicked in—Tammi made a point of connecting with her personally. Seeing that the patient was wearing the T-shirt of a Wisconsin sports team, Tammi mentioned her own family's roots in that state. She told us in reflecting on that connection, "So we were having a whole little Wisconsin talk. And in my head I'm like, 'She didn't need to know.'" What the patient didn't need to know was that she was among the last patients to be seen by Tammi's clinic in Fargo. "She didn't need that emotional labor to know that she's this very profound person to me.' So, I was able to interact with her."

Unbeknownst to the patient and to most people outside of a small circle of confidants, Tammi had been working for months before *Dobbs* on the plan that her husband referred to in their phone call right after the decision. Tammi had suspected what was coming because she had worked in abortion care virtually her entire adult life.

But she didn't grow up committed to being an abortion provider. She grew up in a strongly Catholic family, and as an adolescent considered herself to be pro-life. However, her views began to change when she was in college. Tammi was taking courses in social work and women's studies when a close friend had a traumatic unwanted pregnancy that really affected her. This experience, plus the content of her coursework, led her to understand the importance of reproductive freedom.

After Tammi graduated, one of her professors recommended her for a job in a local abortion clinic in Fargo. In 1993, Tammi began her path down a life of abortion provision with a one-day-a-week job as a patient educator. This caused some tension with Tammi's parents, who remain antiabortion to this day. But they nonetheless do support their daughter. She described how they view the situation: "As practicing Catholics, we cannot support what you do. But you seem to be doing well in your field and we're proud of that."

What her parents are proud of is that Tammi has risen through the ranks at her clinic to become an outspoken and nationally recognized abortion provider. She turned her once-a-week job into a full-time administrator position. Then, when some of the people running this clinic opened a new clinic in Fargo, Tammi moved with them in 1998. Tammi has been with that clinic, Red River Women's Clinic, ever since, working her way up to becoming clinic director and then clinic owner. For over two decades before *Dobbs*, the clinic had been the only abortion-providing facility in North Dakota.

In her role as a clinic owner, Tammi has years and years of experience battling North Dakota to keep the clinic open in the face of antiabortion legislation and hostility. For instance, when we first spoke to her at the beginning of 2022, she was involved in yet another round of litigation against the state, this time about "abortion reversal." North Dakota had passed a law that compelled abortion providers to give their patients false medical information: that a medication abortion could be reversed if the second drug was not taken and if, instead, the patient was given large doses of progesterone. This idea is not supported by any peer-reviewed medical evidence and was wholly concocted by the antiabortion movement.

Tammi and her clinic sued the state over the requirement in 2019, and the litigation had dragged on since then. Tammi told us she was surprised at the state's aggressiveness in the litigation and at the broad scope of the depositions. The state had deposed four of Tammi's frontline staff, which was unusual in these cases: normally a clinic owner or its medical director was the target of depositions. Tammi told us that the staff members, who worked mainly as medical assistants, came out of their depositions with tears in their eyes because of the combative nature of the state's approach.

Tammi knew at the time that there was a much bigger storm cloud on the horizon and had begun working on the plan that would save her clinic. Like many people in the pro-choice movement, Tammi knew the Supreme Court was likely going to overturn *Roe*. According to North Dakota law, if that happened the state's abortion ban would take effect roughly thirty days later. That would mean Red River Women's Clinic would have to close. So Tammi devised a plan to move the clinic without disrupting service for patients.

Fargo is on the far eastern side of the state, on the Red River, which forms the state line between North Dakota and Minnesota. Tammi's plan was to move the clinic just across the river to Moorhead, Minnesota.

Given their proximity, Moorhead and Fargo are almost sister cities. And given the proximity, the move would mean that a new clinic would be only five or ten minutes from the site of the old one. However, that short drive would make all the difference in the world.

In some ways, this new location would be better for the clinic. Not only would it continue to be able to operate just over the river, but in Minnesota, the clinic would be subject to much more abortion-friendly laws, as Minnesota is a considerably more hospitable state for abortion provision than North Dakota. However, Tammi was distraught at the prospect of abandoning North Dakota and leaving the state with no abortion clinic. Geographically it was a small step, but the principle was huge. She told us in early 2022, "I'm not going to do it unless I'm forced to. I will not abandon North Dakota. I will not be the one that makes it so there is not one clinic in this state." With emotion she spoke of "everything we've gone through, everything we've fought for. Damn it, they have tried everything to kick me out of there, and it's not going to happen—unless it is actually illegal to provide care, unless they overturn *Roe v. Wade.*"

Tammi began her real estate search toward the end of 2021, months before *Dobbs*. Although she worked with a professional real estate agent, thanks to the small community of business owners in the area and Tammi's connections from having worked there for decades, she was able to find a suitable property via the local grapevine. A relative of a former employee at Tammi's clinic contacted her to tell her about an available building in Moorhead that could possibly work as a clinic. This tip wasn't a result of pro-choice solidarity; rather, the reason was that the clinic's location in downtown Fargo was near several properties owned by a prominent state politician. The manager of those buildings was having trouble finding tenants because of the presence of protesters at Red River Women's Clinic, so the relative, who worked with the politician's real estate company, told Tammi about the Moorhead property as a way to possibly coax the clinic, and the protesters who gathered there, away from its Fargo site. Tammi also benefited from local networking when it came to negotiating a loan: the banker's sister had formerly worked at the clinic.

As luck would have it, Tammi's own real estate agent had also identified the same building as a possibility. Although the building was larger than the clinic's needs, there were very limited suitable options in Moorhead, so Tammi decided to set in motion its possible purchase. However, she was determined to keep her intentions private for as long as possible, fearing the antiabortion protesters in the area would put pressure on those selling the building and the contractors that Tammi would need to hire. She also feared the possibility of physical danger to the facility. Given the small size of the community of Fargo, Tammi succeeded in keeping her plans private to a remarkable degree, from at the earliest stages of negotiation through the remodeling process and almost until the final move-in date in the summer of 2022. Hoping not to be recognized, she accomplished this feat in part by wearing sunglasses and a large hat on her numerous trips to the property.

In the immediate aftermath of *Dobbs*, the Fargo clinic was able to remain open for several additional weeks, as the North Dakota ban hadn't yet taken effect and court challenges proceeded. As occurred with other abortion facilities across the nation, patients still called the clinic, fearful that abortions were already banned in North Dakota, although that was not the case. Tammi told us that one patient even called wondering whether she could be retroactively prosecuted for having had an abortion.

As deeply upsetting as the Supreme Court's decision was, Tammi found solace in the enormous outpouring of support she received both locally and nationally. She was a frequent interview subject on local and national media, attracting attention to her clinic's plight that drew warm responses. Besides donations and messages of support pouring in, she received numerous offers of concrete assistance. News of her move to Moorhead had now reached the general public, and offers of help included someone offering free solar panels and an attorney and a graphic designer volunteering their services. When we interviewed her in July 2022 she told us, "We had a guy walk in the door yesterday who had a moving truck saying, 'I can help you move.'" In fact, there were so many offers of help that Tammi had to politely thank most people while turning them down, saying, "We are inundated right now. But we'll put you in our folder of offers of help and assistance."

The actual move to the clinic involved seven-day workweeks and long workdays for Tammi, her husband, and trusted clinic supporters. Many of the helpers came from the group of escorts who had been a steady presence for years in front of the Fargo clinic. The most astonishing form of assistance was an online fundraising campaign started by some of the clinic's supporters. They designed the campaign to help pay for the numerous expenses involved with moving to, opening, and operating the new facility. As the random luck of the internet would have it, this campaign went viral in a way no one could have possibly expected. Initially advertised as a campaign to raise $25,000, the campaign passed the million-dollar mark in a matter of just a few weeks. Tammi was stunned and broke into tears as she watched the donations total soar. With this money Tammi was able to move an entire abortion clinic without incurring debt, a shockingly positive development in the wake of *Dobbs*.

The last day at the Fargo site was an emotional one for Tammi. "We certainly didn't tell patients it was the last day," she said. "At the end of the day, we stood around in the downstairs, by the doctor's desk, and realized, 'Holy shit, this is a big deal. We're leaving this behind.' We got pretty teary thinking about Dr. Miks, our first doctor, and thinking that he'd be so proud of us. We just talked about all the memories that we had in the building." After this period of catharsis, Tammi, characteristically, sprang into action. "OK, I got my van. Who wants to help pack up? And everyone helped."

The move to Moorhead opened up a brand-new world to Tammi. In particular, the political environment in Minnesota regarding abortion was starkly different from what Tammi had known for decades in North Dakota. For instance, while working to get her new clinic ready she noticed a call on her cell phone from an unrecognized number. Like many parents upon seeing an unknown number, Tammi feared something had happened to her college-age daughter, so she answered apprehensively. The caller turned out to be Senator Amy Klobuchar, one of Minnesota's two US senators. As Tammi paraphrased the conversation, the senator said, "'Thank you so much for what you are doing. We will do our part. We've got your back.' This would never have happened in North Dakota."

But Minnesota's high-level political delegation wasn't done. Senator Klobuchar's call welcoming Red River Women's Clinic to the state was followed by a visit to the clinic by the state's other US senator, Tina Smith, and several of her staff. (In March 2024, Tammi was a guest of Senator Smith at the State of the Union address.) Then later, in the summer of 2022, Tammi attended a Zoom meeting with Governor Tim Walz and Lieutenant Governor Peggy Flanagan of Minnesota, to which all the abortion providers in the state were invited. Then, Keith Ellison, the Minnesota attorney general, visited the clinic during his fall 2022 election campaign. Closer to home, prior to opening the new facility, Tammi had cordial meetings with the Moorhead chief of police and mayor, the latter even friending her on Facebook.

Moving to Minnesota meant not only friendly politicians but also an end to the need for Red River Women's Clinic to comply with onerous abortion restrictions required by the state. One of the North Dakota laws Tammi was happiest to be done with was the requirement to tell each patient, at the time of her first contact with the clinic, "North Dakota law defines abortion as terminating the life of a whole, separate, unique living human being." What Tammi experienced in Minnesota was almost the exact opposite of North Dakota. In the summer of 2022, shortly before the clinic's move, Minnesota removed a number of its own restrictions, such as a twenty-four-hour waiting period, making abortion provision even more straightforward for providers and patients. Another big gain from the move to Minnesota was that there were a number of other abortion-providing facilities in the state, giving Tammi a local community of peers, something she did not have in North Dakota.

Despite the much more favorable location, Tammi was not able to escape antiabortion protesters. The people who had been a steady presence at the Fargo site soon learned of the Moorhead location and resumed their activity there. On the first day of clinic operations, two of the protesters entered the clinic parking lot, which was the private property of Red River Women's Clinic, and claimed, oddly, that the police had given them permission to be there. Tammi, having already met with the Moorhead police chief, had expected something like this. She called 911, and the police came promptly and ordered the protesters to leave.

More troubling incidents with protesters ensued. At the new location, one of the clinic escorts heard a protester say that escorts "should have their fingers cut off" for helping abortion patients. Another protester was overheard saying something to the effect of "we should bomb this place." The clinic reported both of these incidents to the FBI. A local agent visited the man who mentioned the bomb at his home and ultimately concluded that it was not a viable threat. Besides the local FBI agent, with whom Tammi has dealt in both Fargo and Moorhead, there is an agent in Minneapolis—Tammi refers to this agent as the "repro person" for the state—who stays in touch with all the state's providers to help keep them safe.

BUILDING IN THE MOST UNLIKELY LOCATION

Julie Burkhart was partway through one of the most unlikely responses to the anticipated decision in *Dobbs*—building a new abortion clinic in Casper, Wyoming—when tragedy struck. On May 25, 2022, just weeks after the leak of the *Dobbs* decision on May 2, Julie was awakened very early in the morning: "My phone rang, and it displayed the name of one of our contractors and I thought, 'This is probably going to be a bad phone call.' I was thinking maybe there was a burst pipe, maybe we had a plumbing issue. I certainly didn't think arson." Unfortunately, she was right that it was bad, but she hadn't imagined just how bad.

She was told that her clinic, Wellspring Health Access, which was well on its way to completion before *Dobbs* was expected to be decided, had been firebombed. She quickly went to the clinic, and when she arrived at the site she was devastated to see the extent of the damage. Half to two-thirds of the clinic interior would need to be gutted and rebuilt. Thankfully, Julie's insurance company agreed to pay for the cost of the demolition and rebuilding, reported in the press as $300,000.[1] Julie was crushed, describing it as "a gut punch." But she had already seen the worst the antiabortion movement could possibly throw at her, and this new attack wasn't going to stop her.

Julie's commitment to abortion runs deep. She attributes her identification as a feminist and her career-long devotion to working in abortion to being raised by a second-wave feminist mother. "Bless my mother," she said. "She dragged me to her feminist meetings when I was in grade school. So I grew up hearing the [pro-choice] people talk, and going to these meetings, and probably being bored out of my mind as a child. But this [work] found me. I did not find it."

She started working in the field of abortion provision during college when, in 2001, she took a summer position in a clinic in Wichita, Kansas. After college she took a full-time job at another Wichita abortion clinic, owned and run by George Tiller. Since then, except for a brief foray into managing political campaigns, her entire adult life has been spent working in this field.

Both unfortunately and fortunately, Julie's work with Dr. Tiller prepared her for what she experienced in 2022. The year 2001 was a volatile time in abortion politics. Dr. Tiller had been targeted for years by the national antiabortion movement because he was one of only a handful of abortion providers who performed abortions in the third trimester. His practice's focus on these later abortions offered care mostly for patients whose pregnancies had gone horribly wrong, either because of severe fetal anomalies or because of serious health conditions of the pregnant person. In 1991, a decade before Julie started working with Dr. Tiller, thousands of antiabortion protesters from all over the country had descended on Wichita for the so-called "Summer of Mercy" and laid siege for several months to Dr. Tiller's clinic and several others then operating in Wichita. Then, in 1993, an antiabortion extremist shot Dr. Tiller in both arms.

Julie worked with Dr. Tiller from 2001 until 2009. During that time Dr. Tiller was one of the most polarizing figures in the abortion world. He was reviled by abortion opponents but cherished by the abortion provider community because of his willingness to accept their most difficult cases and to treat these patients with compassion and respect. Julie experienced both the attacks and the love directed at Dr. Tiller firsthand.

She also experienced the unthinkable on May 31, 2009. That morning, Dr. Tiller was serving as an usher in his Wichita church when an antiabortion zealot came into the church and shot Dr. Tiller point-blank in the head, killing him almost instantly. The assassination rocked the abortion world, and Julie still mourns his death to this day.

From her time working at Dr. Tiller's clinic, the immediate aftermath of his murder, and her work since then, Julie realized that she is deeply committed to this work no matter what happens. She credits the enormous influence Dr. Tiller had on her as a mentor. At the time of his death, his was the only abortion facility still in operation in Wichita, and it immediately ceased operations after he was killed. After the assassination Julie contacted Dr. Tiller's widow and arranged to buy the clinic. Eventually she was able to resume abortion care there, though the new clinic did not provide third-trimester care. She also opened new clinics in Oklahoma City and Seattle and adopted one of Dr. Tiller's many slogans, "Trust Women," as the name of the new clinics. Although as of 2022 she was no longer involved with Trust Women clinics, her experience with Dr. Tiller and her commitment to continuing his legacy continues to motivate her.

Because of her decades of experience resisting the violence of the antiabortion movement, the arson in Casper in May 2022, as devastating as it was, did not derail Julie's plans. She had been actively working to open this clinic for over a year. When we first talked with her in early 2022, she told us the idea wasn't hers. Rather, in the summer of 2021, local pro-choice activists had approached her about the possibility of opening a clinic in Casper. At the time there were only two doctors providing abortions in Wyoming, both in Jackson, at the western edge of the state, some 250 miles away, and both offered only medication abortion.

Casper, in the eastern portion of a red state, may seem like an odd choice to establish an abortion clinic, but the local group who approached Julie had its reasons. The core group of about a dozen who advocated for the clinic included an employee of a local abortion fund, a reproductive rights lobbyist, a minister, a city council member, other healthcare providers, and those Julie described as "community activists." The group convinced Julie that Casper was a desirable spot because of its unique location. Casper is a college town, suggesting both that it contains a population of people in the age group most likely to need an abortion and that it is more liberal than most places in the highly conservative state. Also, the planned clinic would hopefully draw patients not only from underserved places in Wyoming but also from neighboring South Dakota, which had virtually no abortion access even prior to *Dobbs*, and Nebraska, which had very limited access as well.

Julie acknowledged in this first interview that opening and sustaining a clinic in such a deeply conservative state was by any measure a long shot—particularly with the threat of a negative *Dobbs* decision looming. Nevertheless, Julie joined forces with the local group and was committed to opening in Casper. She spent late 2021 and early 2022 meeting with community groups and state and local officials. She told us she was aware that, given Wyoming's conservative politics and the Supreme Court's likely ruling in *Dobbs*, there would likely be difficulties ahead, but she expressed the group's consensus that it was imperative to take action before *Dobbs* rather than waiting until after. "We can't afford to sit back and wait," she said. "By doing this right now, hopefully we'll have more power by having the clinic up and running. So if something does happen in Wyoming, we will have that presence. We will have community ties. We will have standing if we have to go to court."

Being ready to go to court weighed heavily on the minds of Julie and her partners. They talked "with a variety of people, looking at the laws that have been passed, and not passed as well, in Wyoming, talking to folks about the Wyoming constitution, where services are and where they are lacking." Ironically, one thing Julie learned early on about Wyoming's constitution was that after the passage of the Affordable Care Act in 2010, which was deeply resented by many in this conservative state, the voters passed an amendment to the state constitution that declared Wyoming citizens had the right to make their own decisions about healthcare. Never in a million years would the drafters of this anti-Obamacare amendment have expected that its existence in the Wyoming constitution would eventually be a key part of Julie's decision to push ahead with an abortion clinic in the face of the Supreme Court's overturning *Roe*. But Julie and her colleagues were buoyed by the prospect that this amendment would be a powerful weapon to keep abortion legal in the state.

Julie also pointed to other unique aspects of Wyoming that made the case for gambling on opening an abortion clinic the year the Supreme Court was set to overrule *Roe*. She cited the state's tradition of libertarianism—a "live and let live" attitude. She also explained that Wyoming had more generous gestational limits than some other states and that the state had no waiting period to get an abortion. She even suggested that opening a clinic in Wyoming was actually easier than in other places because of the state's "Wild West" attitude toward regulatory issues. Because of the state's lax approach to regulation, Julie said, "the beauty of it is we don't have to operate as an ambulatory surgery center." Julie was referring to requirements in some states that abortion clinics have to satisfy that require them to make expensive and medically unnecessary upgrades to their physical plants. In Wyoming, Julie explained that unlike in those states, "we don't have certain rules and regulations."

Not everyone shared Julie's optimistic view of the prospects of opening a clinic in Wyoming. Julie freely acknowledged that some allies in the national pro-choice movement were supportive but skeptical. Lawyers from a national organization that she had worked with in the past were "lukewarm," she said. Though these legal allies wished Julie well, they were not able to devote resources to working with her, presumably because, Julie explained, their resources were committed to working with clinics in other locations with a better chance of success post-*Dobbs*. Julie and a group of supporters had decided to start a nonprofit organization, Wellspring Health Access, that would be the legal operator of the clinic. A different national pro-choice group did eventually help Julie find a local lawyer who agreed to work with her.

The new clinic took a huge step forward when, just before we talked with Julie the first time in 2022, a wealthy donor purchased a suitable building and agreed to let Wellspring Health Access rent the space from her. With the physical location identified, Julie began talking to a number of doctors and nurses who were interested in working at the new clinic. Julie's initial hope was that the clinic could open in June 2022 and that it would offer abortions up to twenty-four weeks, well above the ten-week limit for medication abortions offered by the two doctors in Jackson.

The vision for the new clinic went beyond abortion care. Julie hoped it would become a full-service reproductive health practice—in addition to abortion, the clinic would offer family planning services, general gynecology, and gender-affirming services. In reference to gender-affirming services she said, "We really will have this more inclusive model for the community." She pointed out that there was no Planned Parenthood clinic in Casper, and currently the only way people could get family planning services was through their primary-care doctor—if they had one—or through the local health department, although that option was often unreliable. As for gender-affirming care, Casper has an active LGBTQ community, and representatives of that community had specifically asked that the new clinic include these services.

Renovating the facility was a challenge. Abortion clinics in hostile locations have a history of difficulty in finding and retaining contractors because of local pressure directed at the contractors, who usually do not have the commitment to the issue the clinic does. The building was already zoned for medical use, so Julie "told the contractors that we're a 'women's healthcare clinic,' and we're going to be providing a variety of healthcare for the community at large." Julie was careful never to use the word "abortion" in conversations with contractors. The contractors did eventually learn that the clinic would provide abortion services, but fortunately, they did not abandon the job. They did, however, take care to avoid controversy by choosing not to display a sign at the worksite naming their company, as they otherwise normally would do.

As the building renovations progressed, the political landscape in Wyoming shifted dramatically. In March 2022, the legislature passed and then the governor promptly signed a trigger law stipulating that if *Roe* were to be overturned, almost all abortions in the state would be banned.[2] Nonetheless, Julie proceeded full steam ahead with her dream of opening before *Dobbs* was announced. She was making progress on her plan to hire four doctors, one for each week of the month and had identified several others who could be called upon on an as-needed basis. She had an agreement with a Pacific Northwest physician with whom she had previously worked extensively to be the clinic's medical director and had hired other staff as well. With staffing set, Julie set an opening date for the clinic in mid-June, feeling excited that this would likely occur before *Dobbs* was announced.

But then the arsonist struck, and all of Julie's plans were derailed. What made the arson particularly unfortunate is that even in the event of *Dobbs*'s overturning *Roe*, Julie would have been able to keep the clinic open because of the other services it planned to offer. Like others, Julie was devastated by *Dobbs*. She described her reaction that day: "I was so angry, so angry, anger and hurt. I've now spent my career in this field, and looking back at that, and just everything that everybody's done and fought for, and all the good things, and just continuing to try to hold the line and push the needle, and then blink of an eye, it's gone. It just made me feel so sad for everybody who's invested all these years and energy." Julie spent the day after the decision listening to music with the volume turned up— including old feminist anthems from the 1970s.

Despite the setback Julie was still committed to making abortion accessible in conservative states. Speaking more passionately than in other interviews, she said immediately after *Dobbs* was decided, "I want to tell you in Wyoming, we are going to litigate, we are going to fight this thing to the end, and we're going to see . . . if we can hold the line there."

Julie and her allies had begun planning a litigation strategy in spring 2022. Wellspring Health Access, the two abortion providers from Jackson, a few Wyoming physicians, and several others from the core group supporting the clinic joined forces to bring a lawsuit in state court challenging the trigger ban. They were joined by a Jewish law student at the University of Wyoming who brought a claim against the abortion ban arguing that it violated their religious freedom, a legal strategy that is also being tried in several other states.[3]

Immediately after *Dobbs*, their litigation met with success. The state district court judge granted a temporary restraining order and a preliminary injunction, which prevented the ban from going into effect on July 27, the day it had been scheduled to do so. This was a huge victory, though tempered by Wellspring's being unable to take advantage of the ruling because of post-fire construction work. However, the other doctors in Jackson were able to continue offering abortions for patients.

As the year progressed Julie focused on rebuilding the clinic, including building a new fence and upgrading security in other ways. The good news was that her insurance had covered most of the repairs. The bad news was that her insurance company sent her a notice of cancellation, a frequent occurrence for abortion clinics that are attacked. Fortunately one of her team was able to secure new coverage, but not without the situation being a "real headache" for everyone involved.

At the end of 2022, the investigation into the arson was a source of frustration for Julie. At the beginning of the investigation, she said, the local police and federal officials had been appropriately responsive. The police actively solicited video footage from nearby businesses, as well as having access to Wellspring's own video cameras. The federal Bureau of Alcohol, Tobacco and Firearms (ATF) had posted a reward for information leading to the arrest of the perpetrator. A state representative even reached out to her about the arson, offering sympathy, but no concrete plan of assistance.

However, when we asked Julie if she felt law enforcement was doing enough, she demurred. She acknowledged they were "nice, responsive people" but feared they didn't understand the unique issues connected to antiabortion violence. She hoped to bring in experts in antiabortion violence to meet with all the agencies involved in investigating the arson attack. This had worked well for Julie previously in Kansas and Oklahoma. She hoped that bringing together the US attorney, the local police department, federal marshals, the FBI, the ATF, and movement experts to have "a big roundtable discussion" would move the investigation forward and make everyone more accountable. Eventually her efforts to move things along had an impact: the arsonist was arrested in March 2023 and then pled guilty four months later and was sentenced to five years in prison.[4]

The post-*Dobbs* period also brought good news for the clinic's opening. In November 2022, the state judge hearing the clinic's lawsuit continued the injunction against the ban, and as of June 2024, the litigation challenging the law was still ongoing. In the meantime, with the law held up in court, Julie was finally able to open her doors in April 2023, almost a full year after both the arson and *Dobbs*.

Antiabortion sentiment swirling around the clinic has not dissipated, though. Shortly after the clinic opened, the mayor of Casper posted an image of a man dancing in fire in response to a media post about the clinic. Many in the community felt this was a call to violence and worried about a reprise of the 2022 attack. The mayor ultimately apologized but refused to delete the image.[5] Wellspring's provision of gender-affirming care has also become a flash point—protesters have called on the city council to ban this service.

At the end of the momentous year of 2022, before the clinic was even able to open and start seeing patients, Julie was dealing with a clinic that had been set on fire, a state legislature that had made clear it would try to ban nearly all abortions, protesters who showed up weekly at the clinic construction site, and litigation whose outcome was uncertain. But this big gamble paid off, as Wellspring Health Access opened to patients in spring 2023, expanding access for those in Wyoming, even in the face of *Dobbs*.

FLYING PATIENTS FOR CARE

In many ways, it was a fantastical proposal. In late 2021, a group of clergy approached Curtis Boyd, the owner and medical director of two abortion clinics in Texas and New Mexico, about flying patients from Texas to New Mexico to receive abortion care after the sixth week of pregnancy. Patients would be accompanied by a member of the clergy and arrive back home in Texas later the same day. To those who didn't know Curtis, probably nothing about this makes sense. Clergy helping abortion patients? An abortion provider devising a plan to fly patients? And patients going to this length to get an abortion? But to Curtis, everything about this plan made sense . . . except for one thing—the political landscape that necessitated its creation.

Curtis Boyd's involvement with provision began in the 1960s, so he has seen and experienced almost everything there is to see in abortion provision. As a young doctor in 1968 he started providing illegal abortions. He ultimately performed thousands, first in a small Texas town, later in Dallas, and eventually in New Mexico. Like many doctors providing this necessary but, pre-*Roe*, illegal care, his abortion provision took place under the auspices of the Clergy Consultation Service, a group of Protestant and Jewish clergy who set up a referral service for women seeking abortions before *Roe* made abortion legal throughout the country.

Curtis's commitment to providing care even though it was illegal stemmed from taking his ethical and moral obligations as a physician seriously. Though the notorious "back alley butchers" of the pre-*Roe* era dominate public perceptions of the typical abortion provider of that era, Curtis is a prime example of what one of us in previous writing has termed "doctors of conscience"—physicians whose illegal provision was not motivated primarily by money or because they were incapable of succeeding in a mainstream medical practice, but rather because they were moved by the desperation of women with unwanted pregnancies.[6]

Curtis's commitment was combined with his religious faith. He came from a deeply religious family and was himself ordained as a Baptist preacher while still in his teens. Later, while a medical student, he became involved with the far more liberal Unitarian church, as well as the various social justice movements of the 1960s. His immersion in these two overlapping circles cemented his commitment to abortion work. This background made his teaming up with the Clergy Consultation Service in the late 1960s a natural fit.

Curtis has continued to team with clergy throughout his almost sixty-year career as an abortion provider and clinic owner. Prior to *Dobbs* he ran two very busy abortion clinics, one in Dallas and the other in Albuquerque. A group of ministers had for some time been coming to Curtis's Dallas clinic to offer spiritual counseling to patients who wished it, and this group first proposed the travel idea to Curtis in late 2021.

These were the first months of SB8's implementation in Texas. Because this law prohibited abortions after six weeks, the patient volume of the Dallas clinic had significantly decreased as only a fraction of the usual 200 to 250 patients per week were able to seek care within the six-week limit. Seeing numerous women being turned away because of the new law, one of the members of the clergy group proposed a way to bring groups of patients to Curtis's Albuquerque clinic. The initial idea was to have the patients take an overnight bus trip, but eventually the clergy came up with the idea of buying group airline tickets in advance—it would be both cheaper and more efficient. They proposed this idea to Curtis; being committed to doing whatever it takes to get women the care they need, he was on board.

The details of the plan came together quickly. As it originally operated, eligible low-income patients met at a local church and traveled together to the Dallas airport, accompanied by a minister. The size of the group could be anywhere from ten to twenty-five. Curtis explained to us the rationale for their being accompanied: "Some of these women have never been in an airport, let alone a plane. And it can be intimidating. They get lost, and they don't make it to their gate on time." The minister's presence helped keep everyone calm and made the process flow more easily.

Once the group landed in Albuquerque, other religious supporters stepped in. Staff from the New Mexico chapter of the Religious Coalition for Reproductive Choice met the group and accompanied them in a rented bus to the clinic. Curtis described the flow of the day: "They get there at midmorning. We do the procedures from midmorning to midafternoon. And we provide them with the medication they need, food while they're there to eat after they've finished, and then they go back. So, this is one day, they leave Dallas in the morning, and they're back home that evening."

In light of his background as a Baptist preacher, it's not surprising that Curtis was particularly gratified by the involvement with the ministers in this program. He told us, "It's a powerful symbolic issue. When everyone's thinking, 'Well, if you're religious, you're antiabortion. If you're for abortion, you must not believe in God. You're not a good Christian.' What we want is to counter that and say, 'Look, these are ordained ministers, chaplains. They believe in your right. They want to help you. They are going as shepherds, if you will.'"

When the program first started in late 2021, Curtis's staff at the Dallas clinic started the patient's care there, carrying out various aspects of the patients' pre-abortion care—counseling, ultrasonography, lab work, charting—and then transmitted this information to the sister New Mexico clinic. All of the Texas patients were at twelve weeks' gestation age or less, and initially they were offered medication abortions.

Even though he was proud of the way he was able to offer patients this care despite the Texas law, when he took a step back Curtis recognized the absurdity of the lengths that these patients had to go to in order to take a pill. He said, "I give them a mifepristone pill and a glass of water. Then I say to them, 'That's it, you flew all the way from Dallas for that! I'm sorry you had to go through this.'" Though the second medication in the abortion pill regimen, misoprostol, is typically taken twenty-four hours after the mifepristone, out of an abundance of legal caution so that no one could claim the abortion was completed in Texas—the clinic told the patients to take the misoprostol pills while still in New Mexico.

After *Dobbs*, Curtis continued this program but had to change procedures. His Dallas clinic had shut down patient care, so the pre-abortion workups had to take place in New Mexico rather than Texas. Curtis acknowledged that he had become more concerned about legal threats from the state of Texas since *Dobbs*. He and his clergy partners worried that their travel program might be considered "aiding and abetting" under the state's complete abortion ban or under SB8. In fact, Curtis stopped the travel program for a short period of time while he and his colleagues consulted with an attorney to sort out the unclarified legal issues the program raised. Curtis then resumed the program, and it was still in operation at the end of 2023. Now, when eligible Texas residents contact the Albuquerque clinic, they are told of the possibility of clergy accompaniment to New Mexico. Unitarian ministers meet the patients at the Dallas–Fort Worth airport, and Religious Coalition for Reproductive Choice representatives continue to greet the travelers upon their arrival in New Mexico.

The travel program, which ceased operation in 2024 when Curtis sold the Albuquerque clinic, was not the only way Curtis prepared for *Dobbs*. Like so many others, he was confident that the Supreme Court was going to overrule *Roe*, which would mean that patients would flock to his New Mexico clinic but that his Texas clinic would have to close. Accordingly, he began to explore the possibility of building a large new clinic in Albuquerque to replace his current building. He had originally hoped to open it in late 2023, but because other abortion providers expanded in Albuquerque due to the flood of patients into New Mexico, as 2023 dawned, Curtis decided to remain in his current building.

When we talked with Curtis at the end of 2022, the need for focusing on New Mexico was evident because of the effect of Texas's abortion ban. The week immediately after Texas's ban went into effect, he said, "In Albuquerque, it was chaos. I think we had over eight hundred calls from Texas. We only know that because [our phone system] records the number of calls. We couldn't possibly answer the phone, let alone see all of them." Curtis's staff was booking patients three or four weeks out because of the huge increase in volume.

Curtis noticed an interesting irony of the frantic rush in New Mexico. The difficulties that so many patients, from both states with bans and states where abortion remained legal, had in scheduling abortions has led to a very high no-show rate. Speaking sympathetically of the people who have been scheduled several weeks out but then don't show up for their appointment, Curtis explained that many keep looking for earlier abortion appointments at other clinics. He explained further about a hypothetical patient: "She starts calling and trying to find someplace else to go. She goes wherever she can go. So, it's chaotic. And it's frustrating. And what we are faced with, and I'm sure other places are too, is ending up with unused appointment time."

Looking to the other side of the country, to make up for the expected loss of his Texas clinic, in 2022 Curtis purchased a highly regarded abortion clinic in West Palm Beach, Florida that was established a few years after *Roe*. The logic of buying the Florida facility was to better serve pregnant people in the South, where it was clear that Alabama, Mississippi, Tennessee, and Louisiana, and possibly other states would ban abortion if *Roe* fell.

By the end of 2022, though, Curtis admitted that the purchase of the Florida clinic may have been a mistake. Speaking of the state's increasingly conservative legislature he said, "They can do anything they want." Moreover, commenting on the Florida governor's long-term national ambitions, he said with frustration, "I didn't realize [Governor Ron] DeSantis was going to go off the rails." Indeed, months after we last talked with Curtis, in April 2023, despite the state already having passed a fifteen-week abortion ban that at the time had been held up in state court, Governor DeSantis signed a measure banning abortions after six weeks, which took effect in May 2024.

Given his long career in this field, it was impossible for Curtis to describe what he was doing in 2022 in the wake of *Dobbs* without speaking in depth about his feelings regarding the current political environment and its resulting upheaval in his life's work. He ranged from sadness to anger to guarded optimism in how he talked about this moment. In particular, his voice welled with sadness as he described the "devastating" moment of having to close his Dallas clinic because of *Dobbs*. Comparing the loss of the clinic to the death of a friend, he said, "You're waiting for them to die, and you know they're going to die. But at the actual moment that they take their last breath, it's very emotional. That's when they're dead. So, it was somewhat like that. We knew it was going to happen. We tried to prepare the staff that it's going to happen. So when it happened there was a great deal of mourning and crying."

He reflected on what he had been through as a Texas abortion provider for more than half a century: "We did incredible work. The staff was outstanding. To lose that? I went from a little house in Texas"—the first building where he provided illegal abortions with the Clergy Counseling Service in 1968—"and it's been a continuous operation since that time. We had . . . fifty years of really solid progress. Fifty years. And not that it was easy. It got really hard [with] the protesters. We went through arsons, death threats, invasions, but we never [thought of leaving] the state of Texas."

Curtis has no plans to return to providing illegal abortions, saying, "I'm going to provide abortions where I can. Now, I'm eighty-five years old. I don't want to spend the last ten years of my life in prison, quite frankly." He predicted that relatively few doctors would perform illegal abortions in this new era. Referring to the likely response of antiabortion law enforcement officials to anyone found doing so, he said, "They will go after you with a vengeance."

In assessing the current moment in which there is no longer a national constitutional right to abortion, Curtis turned to a theme that has motivated him throughout his long career—the unfair treatment of women in American society. "What this is for me is a loss for women," he said. "Yes, it is about abortion, but that's not the primary thing for me. This is a loss of women's rights of their equality, and their liberty promised them under the Constitution. This is about women, in general. Whether you favor or oppose abortion, you should oppose the restriction of a woman to be able to make her own decision regarding her life and body."

LUCK AND HOPE

Tammi, Julie, and Curtis know that they've benefitted from fortuitous circumstances in their ability to respond creatively to *Dobbs*—location, supporters, funding, coupled with their passion and hard work. For now they've come through with creative solutions to the problems created by *Dobbs*, solutions that have maintained and even expanded access despite the overturning of *Roe*.

Tammi told us that she knows she is lucky to be in this situation even after the Supreme Court ruled and her home state banned abortion. She never would have imagined that her story would be one of the most successful post-*Dobbs* transitions out of a state with an abortion ban to a state without one. A combination of factors made the move from Fargo, North Dakota, to Moorhead, Minnesota, not only possible but seemingly as smooth as could be hoped for: Tammi's prodigious energy, the clinic's location near the state line, her highly visible local and national profile, a seemingly endless well of supporters, and an internet fundraiser going viral and drawing massive donations from across the country. In fact, Tammi admitted to us that she had some form of survivor's guilt when she thought about how many of her comrades elsewhere in the close-knit provider community were not able to have such a positive outcome after the fall of *Roe*.

Despite her own successful move, Tammi is left with deep anger over North Dakota now being left without a clinic. She described where this entire move has left her. "I love this facility better. I am so much happier in a one-level building, with a parking lot, without the restrictions that we had to have in North Dakota. But there are some days I'm just like, 'They fucking won.' You know? And that's what pisses me off."

Julie's experience and determination put a different spin on this new landscape. It is no surprise that the journalist Eyal Press, writing in the *Nation*, has called Julie "a poster child for moral courage."[7] And it's also no surprise that, in explaining to us why she persisted, Julie answered, "I have faith. I'm going with my gut here. But we'll see." Even if Wellspring Health Access ultimately has to close because Wyoming's abortion ban takes effect, Julie is confident that she's doing the right thing. "I think about Oklahoma, you know?" she said, referring to when the state banned abortion after *Dobbs*. "We provided healthcare to people in Oklahoma City for six years. And I think about the literally thousands of people who came in our doors there and at least we had six years to help them. That's worth it. So that's the way I'm approaching Wyoming."

Curtis's faith has translated into a somewhat surprising long-term outlook. Looking to the future of reproductive freedom, despite deep disappointment over *Dobbs*, Curtis retains some optimism. He was buoyed by the electoral backlash to the decision that has been evident across the country. And he continues to believe that ultimately those who support abortion will triumph over those who oppose it. He proclaimed, "It's going to be a long time and hard to overcome. Now, we will eventually win. That's what gives me hope in my old age. I don't think I'm going to necessarily see that, but I have confidence because we have the majority, a good majority. And eventually, we'll get ourselves organized and prevail. What I really hope is that this Supreme Court has kicked the hornet's nest."

Each of these providers here, along with others like them in other parts of the country, faced *Dobbs* and took creative steps to continue to provide care to patients. They go a long way to explain why abortion numbers have not dropped precipitously because of abortion bans but in fact have slightly increased. Unknowingly summing up the new situation for the three providers featured in this chapter as well as many others, Tammi told a journalist, speaking of her foes, "I don't think they actually anticipated that this is what the outcome would be. That we'd actually be in a better place and just serve all the same people."[8]

CHAPTER FOUR

PIVOT MASTERS

We're in a chess game and we haven't gotten checkmate. We're doing check, check, check, check. Unfortunately, we're doing check, check, check with pregnant people and their families' lives.

—KARRIE GALLOWAY,
Planned Parenthood Association of Utah

The phrase "the cruelty is the point" came into wide use during Donald Trump's presidency.[1] Now it has carried into the post-*Roe* world in reference to the extraordinary hardships imposed on pregnant women who have been denied essential care. Whether it's people facing pregnancy emergencies who cannot get the help they need at hospitals or people no longer wanting to be pregnant for other reasons who can't get an abortion at a clinic that used to be in their state, being denied care that they would have gotten before *Dobbs* is, simply, cruel.

Additionally, a new twist on that phrase has arisen since the Supreme Court overturned *Roe*: "The chaos is the point." Several commentators have used these words to describe the post-*Roe* landscape. Because everything about this new environment has been wrapped up in legalese that seems to change by the day while leaving many questions unresolved, people are confused, and that confusion itself is a form of harm. Individuals' need to get an abortion has become a story of constantly changing circumstances as they encounter a plethora of unclear legal minutiae and jargon: trigger bans, territorial bans, overlapping restrictions, temporary restraining orders, preliminary injunctions, emergency stays, preemption, third-party standing, arbitrary and capricious, administrative agency law, extraterritoriality, and more.

Whereas before *Roe* was overturned people had to ask themselves whether they wanted to get an abortion, how they were going to pay for it, and where the closest clinic was, now the questions are different: Is it legal to get an abortion where I live? If so, can I get an abortion if I'm past twenty weeks in pregnancy? Past fifteen weeks? Past six weeks? Are abortion pills available or do I have to get a procedure? Can I travel to get an abortion, and if so, is there going to be a legal issue when I return home? Making matters worse is that the answers to these questions might change from one day to the next.

Abortion providers and helpers have a whole new set of questions as well. Is this patient's condition serious enough for me to be able to provide her an abortion within one of the exceptions under my state law? How do I reconcile a federal law that requires me to care for someone who is pregnant and needs emergency care with my state's law that bans abortion? Can I give abortion pills to this patient from another state that bans abortion even if the patient may travel back home to take the second set of pills? If my state now bans abortion, can I refer callers to clinics in other states? Can I drive patients from a state that bans abortion to a state that doesn't? Can I fund their travel from one state to another?

Providing quality care to patients amid this chaos and confusion has been both the mission and challenge for the three providers featured in this chapter. Providers in all states after *Dobbs* have faced some of these questions. For instance, a provider in a state with an abortion ban still has to think about referrals and exceptions. And a provider in a state that continues to allow abortion, maybe even affirmatively supporting abortion rights and access, needs to think about caring for patients who travel and also about any national-level changes concerning the administration of abortion pills.

The providers featured in this chapter have had to deal with uncertainty and chaos almost since the moment *Dobbs* was decided. Their states have gone back and forth with their laws about abortion, sometimes because of court decisions, other times because of legislative policy changes. The policy whiplash has been exacerbated by a number of unanswered questions that increase the chaos and confusion. Through it all, these providers have tried to foreground their patients and staff to make sure patients get the best care possible without staff putting themselves at legal risk. It has been exhausting to practice in this environment, but abortion has continued in the three providers' states because so far they have been able to continue to provide quality care to their patients, even though *Roe* has fallen and even though state officials have tried to make it difficult and confusing.

LENGTHY COURT CHALLENGES

Overruling *Roe* did not mean the end of courts deciding abortion cases. Rather, state courts became more of a focus for abortion litigation. Federal courts have not disappeared from the abortion legal landscape entirely, though, as they continue to hear cases, including two Supreme Court cases decided in June 2024. The first of those, an antiabortion challenge to the FDA's approval of mifepristone, the first drug in a two-drug regimen for medication abortion, was dismissed for procedural reasons. The second also avoided a ruling on the merits, as the Supreme Court decided that it had improperly agreed to hear a case about whether state laws that ban abortion in all circumstances other than when the woman's life is threatened are trumped by the federal law requiring hospitals to stabilize any patient who presents to the emergency room, including a pregnant patient who is facing a medical emergency and whose treatment may require an abortion.[2]

But state courts, which have been hearing and deciding abortion cases for decades without receiving the same attention as the federal courts, have now moved to the forefront. They are the reason that pre-*Dobbs* predictions of almost half of the states banning abortion have not yet come to fruition. State bans on abortion have been halted, either temporarily or for longer, in state courts in Wyoming, Utah, Arizona, Ohio, Iowa, and South Carolina.

While the general public watches these developments from afar, celebrating decisions that go their way and cursing those that don't, those who have to work on the ground in the wake of these decisions don't have that luxury. Instead they have to plan for the various possibilities that arise from the cases while consulting with lawyers about their options. Then, when the decision comes, they have to let everyone know about the change and then implement it for staff and patients. In the crazed fallout from *Dobbs*, this has meant constantly pivoting depending on what courts do and say. Two of the providers we interviewed over the course of 2022, Kwajelyn Jackson in Georgia and Karrie Galloway in Utah, exemplify what providers in states with shifting landscapes have gone through after *Dobbs*.

For four weeks after the Supreme Court overturned *Roe*, Kwajelyn Jackson's clinic in Atlanta, Georgia, was at the epicenter of abortion care in the South. Founded in 1976 as part of a group of feminist abortion clinics, Feminist Women's Health Center had long been seeing traveling abortion patients coming from other Southern states. Before *Dobbs*, Georgia law allowed abortion through twenty-two weeks in pregnancy, so many people in the Deep South who lived in states with earlier gestational limits or without clinics that provided care later in pregnancy traveled to Atlanta. Feminist Women's was one of several Atlanta clinics that saw these patients.

Kwajelyn saw this all coming. Having worked at the clinic for almost a decade, she was now its executive director. Her background provided the perfect mix for this unique time. She moved to Atlanta from St. Louis to attend Spelman College, where she was immersed in Black feminist theory and activism. After college she pursued a career in finance but became disillusioned with her field during the economic collapse of 2008. She quit and transitioned into the nonprofit world, starting as an unpaid intern at an arts nonprofit. There she did everything she could to connect with Atlanta's progressive social justice organizations and learn about the nonprofit world. She eventually became a paid employee, managing an arts center and coordinating volunteers.

After a couple of years in that position, Kwajelyn decided it was time for a change. She had become familiar with Feminist Women's Health Center because of its presence at some of the performance spaces she worked with. She also had been schooled in reproductive justice by, as Kwajelyn called it, "osmosis" through her mother. Kwajelyn's mother had worked for the Planned Parenthood affiliate in St. Louis for several years, doing their sex education programming and internal diversity work. She had exposed Kwajelyn to several of the reproductive justice movement's defining spaces, including the Let's Talk About Sex conference sponsored by the famed reproductive justice group Sister Song, and the group's headquarters, "the Motherhouse." Kwajelyn saw the "through line" of her mother's influence and her time at Spelman as providing her with "a Black feminist foundation to draw from that worldview and analysis" in her next venture: applying for and then being offered the job of volunteer coordinator at Feminist Women's in 2013.

At Feminist Women's, Kwajelyn quickly moved into coordinating, then managing, the clinic's advocacy programs. After Kwajelyn spent four years in that department, the clinic's executive director retired earlier than expected. Already in a leadership position at the clinic, Kwajelyn became the co–interim executive director in 2017 and eventually, after a year in the interim position, became the executive director in 2018. She's been in that position ever since.

Throughout a time of transition such as 2022 after *Roe* had been overturned, Kwajelyn's background proved ideal. As she remarked, "It is fascinating to me that these things came together. My finance stuff, my public policy stuff, and then my mother's social justice work, with a Black feminist foundation. All of those things converged in a way that make me equipped for this role." It also helped that Kwajelyn is an optimist. She told us during our conversations that "abortion will come around again"; even at the end of the rough year that was 2022, she was "confident that if we continue to move in the direction we're moving, that we will survive."

Kwajelyn spent her first several years in her leadership position making sure systems were in place to ensure the organization was being run in a way that was financially sound and ethical. So when 2022 came and the threat to legal abortion became real, she approached it the same way she had approached everything else in her work: paying keen attention to caring for patients within the confines of the law, making sure that her staff was treated well, and ensuring the organization's financial stability through uncertainty and chaos.

Continuing to provide abortion services was tested initially in the month following *Dobbs*. In July, Georgia continued to allow abortion up until twenty-two weeks while the fate of its six-week ban was being decided in the courts. During that time the clinic's volume doubled. Most of the patients continued to be from Georgia, but an increasing number came from states across the South where abortion was almost immediately banned. In particular, Alabama and Tennessee patients flooded the clinic, but patients also came from more distant Southern states like Mississippi, Louisiana, Texas, Arkansas, and Oklahoma. But because Kwajelyn and her staff were able to plan and prepare for this influx, they were able to accommodate the patients who came to the clinic.

What worried Kwajelyn the most was her staff's well-being throughout this "super-intense" period of time. The clinic had to expand its hours for abortions during that period and had some of its highest daily numbers of procedural abortions ever. On one of the days they maxed out at fifty abortions in a day. That day there was one doctor at the clinic who performed all of the abortions over the course of an expanded fourteen-hour day. Because of the overwhelming numbers, the clinic bought dinner for all of the staff who stayed that night to care for the patients. But Kwajelyn knew that this number could not become the norm. "Thirty, maybe thirty-five is manageable with our staff," she told us, "but fifty is too many."

During this time the clinic also saw a huge increase in medication abortion. Medication abortion, the two-drug regimen that was the subject of one of the two abortion-related Supreme Court cases decided in 2024, is usually only used in the first ten to twelve weeks of pregnancy. On the reason for the increase in medication abortion, Kwajelyn said, "It's hard to say what people's decision-making is like, but what I'm imagining, based on people's behavior, is that once they even suspect that they're pregnant, they're not waiting around to sort of toil over it. They're just like, 'I just need to get this done as soon as I can because I might not be able to later.'" And so they ask for a medication abortion.

Kwajelyn had thought this new higher volume would last at least through mid-August. When we talked with her two weeks after *Dobbs* was decided, Kwajelyn had expected litigation over Georgia's six-week ban, passed in 2019, to give her about a two-month buffer. The law had been enjoined in federal court and never took effect because of *Roe*. With *Roe* overruled, everyone in Georgia expected the federal courts to lift the injunction, but it would take time. The federal appeals court had given the parties in the case challenging the 2019 ban three weeks after *Dobbs* to file their papers, and then any decision from the appeals court was expected to go into effect twenty-eight days later. Even with an immediate decision from the appeals court, Kwajelyn and her colleagues had initially thought August 15 would be the earliest the six-week ban would go into effect.

But even the best-laid plans sometimes get disrupted, and that's what happened at the appeals court. When Kwajelyn updated us at the end of 2022, she told us that the court ruled, as expected, that with *Roe* overturned, the six-week ban was constitutional. Pressed by the state of Georgia to implement its order immediately, the federal appeals court set aside the normal process of waiting twenty-eight days for its decision to take effect and reinstated the six-week ban the same day as its decision, July 20.

This was several weeks before Kwajelyn had anticipated, so she and her staff had to act fast: "We really quickly shifted. And fortunately, the day that the injunction was lifted was not an abortion day; it was a Wednesday, so we had a couple of days to get ourselves together and call patients and cancel people, and change our forms. And update our [state-required informed-consent] language and all that stuff. We were able to adjust really quickly and we haven't had any down days in between the shifts in the law. It's not a hard-and-fast six weeks to the day, the way that our law is written. So, we were seeing patients up to the point at which, as the law says, cardiac activity is detectable."

The sudden change of care as a result of the court's decision meant that patients now had a window of only a couple of weeks to get an abortion after realizing they were pregnant instead of several months, resulting in a "steep drop-off" in patient numbers for Feminist Women's. Kwajelyn told us that the clinic was seeing about half of its pre-*Dobbs* volume, which is roughly one-quarter of its volume in the month immediately following *Dobbs* (because the rush from other states had doubled the clinic's volume in that period). In raw numbers, this meant the clinic was caring for about ten to twelve patients a day.

A curious thing happened over this period of time, though. The clinic's numbers began to "constantly continue to creep back up." Kwajelyn was seeing what other states with six-week bans have seen: after some initial shock and confusion about the new law, patients start making decisions earlier in pregnancy to have an abortion.[3] This "new paradigm," as Kwajelyn called it, changed people's behavior. They slowly began to understand the law and then made quicker decisions as a result. Also, Kwajelyn has noticed that with the attention paid to abortion nationally after *Dobbs*, more people coming to her clinic are aware of early-pregnancy medication abortion as an option.

A third factor that came into play was that Georgia's law has exceptions for survivors of rape or incest and cases of fatal fetal anomaly. Even though such cases are few and far between, Feminist Women's has been able to effectively care for these women because, as Kwajelyn explained, "it is important that we are able to be a place that people can go in these situations." With all of these factors at play, by the end of 2022, the clinic's numbers were approaching over twenty cases per abortion day.

After the initial influx followed by the sudden drop in patients, Kwajelyn thought the post-*Dobbs* landscape had stabilized for her clinic. She was wrong. In July, after the federal appeals court had allowed the six-week ban to go into effect, Feminist Women's and several other Georgia clinics and reproductive justice organizations filed a new lawsuit challenging the state's ban. The plaintiffs claimed in this case brought in Georgia state court that the ban violated several different parts of the state constitution. The Georgia judge heard testimony in October and on November 15 ruled that the six-week ban needed to be put on hold.

In the judge's short opinion, he did not rule on whether the ban vi-olated the state constitutional provisions at stake in the case. Rather, he ruled that because the law was enacted in 2019, "when the supreme law of this land unequivocally was—and had been for nearly half a century—that laws unduly restricting abortion before viability were unconstitutional," the law could not spring back into existence now. He based this decision on a Georgia doctrine that if a law is unconstitutional, it is "forever void." Because the six-week ban was unconstitutional when it was enacted in 2019, it "did not become the law of Georgia when it was enacted and it is not the law of Georgia now." If the legislature wants a six-week ban now that the Supreme Court has overruled *Roe*, the judge ruled that it has to pass a new law and not rely on the law that was passed at a time when it was unconstitutional.[4]

For the second time in a matter of months, a court ruling caused Femi-nist Women's to change how late it would perform abortions. Now it could see more people because Georgia's law permitting abortions until twenty-two weeks had once again become the controlling rule. Kwajelyn's staff got on the phone and began calling people to let them know. "We called people that we had previously turned away. We changed our website. We did what we could to try to make sure that people knew, and people came." The decision came on a Tuesday, and the following weekend, the clinic brought in additional doctors to see the influx of patients.

This lasted just over a week. Eight days after the decision halting the six-week ban and a day before Thanksgiving, the Georgia Supreme Court put the lower court judge's decision on hold, thus making the clinic adjust how late in pregnancy it would care for patients for the third time since *Dobbs*. Kwajelyn gave the following statement to the press: "It is cruel that our patients' ability to access the reproductive healthcare they need has been taken away yet again. For the second time this year, we are be-ing forced to turn away those in need of abortion care beyond six weeks of pregnancy. This ban has wreaked havoc on Georgians' lives, and our patients deserve better. We will keep fighting to protect our patients and their health."[5]

The clinic had been prepared, though. Counselors had told patients that the law was in flux and that the clinic would confirm their appoint-ments because everything could have changed between the time the pa-tients' visit was scheduled and the actual visits. Unfortunately for some patients, that's exactly what happened—everything changed. Because of yet another court ruling, they were unable to get the care they would have been able to get just days before.

This case isn't yet finished, so Kwajelyn may once again have to change the clinic's gestational limits because of a court decision. The Georgia Supreme Court reversed the lower court ruling in October 2023 and allowed the state's ban to remain in effect. However, the case will continue in the lower court where the challengers can present other arguments under the state constitution.

When the case is ultimately concluded, the clinic will have to respond, and its patients will have to adjust. If the courts give their final stamp of approval to the six-week ban, Kwajelyn thinks the Georgia legislature will stop there. "I don't think the legislature wants anymore smoke. It would be a knock-down, drag-out fight to go for a total ban. I just don't think they will. I could be wrong, but I think it's highly unlikely that Georgia will go hard for a total ban."

This kind of back-and-forth has been very hard on patients. Kwajelyn said her staff is working really hard to make things as clear as possible to people who call the clinic, but it's "been really difficult." Patients are confused, she said, "I think that there are people who think that abortion is completely illegal, because they don't really understand what's happening. Or they think that because the six-week ban is in effect, a bunch of clinics are closed that are not closed. Which is also confusing. I think the general public is not paying as much attention as we are." Kwajelyn and her staff are "trying to get information out as much as we can through the channels that we can. But I don't think it permeates every community in the same way. So, I do worry about the flow of information and what people know and believe."

With the six-week ban in place and more patients coming in for earlier abortions than expected, Feminist Women's was doing better than anticipated, but the numbers are not quite financially sustainable for the clinic. Even though by the end of 2022 the clinic was seeing more patients, earlier abortions weren't bringing in as much money as later abortions, so there was still a financial gap to keep clinic operations sustainable. To fill the gap, Kwajelyn and her staff had already been planning on expanding their clinic's services. When we talked with her in early 2022, Kwajelyn explained to us that she was exploring fundraising opportunities that were available to her because Feminist Women's is a nonprofit clinic. Although her clinic saw a big uptick in donations post-*Dobbs*, she knew that she couldn't count indefinitely on higher donations because "rage and fear donations" don't last forever.

So instead of relying on fundraising to fill the financial gap, the clinic began focusing on expanding its other services. Feminist Women's has always provided more than just abortion for its clients. A substantial portion of the care it provides is basic gynecological wellness services such as office visits, Pap smears, sexually transmitted infection testing, contraception, HIV treatment, and more. The clinic also has been developing and expanding health services for transgender people. Given the financial landscape with the six-week ban in place, the clinic was considering other expansions— prenatal care, birthing, fertility care, gender-affirming surgery.

Figuring out, as Kwajelyn explained to us, "what the mix is that gets us enough kinds of services at enough price point that gets us closer to" sustainability is the challenge. When we pointed out that her background in finance, policy, and social justice was perfect preparation for this task, Kwajelyn was humble but agreed. "I think so. I think that background really does help me. I know how to read a financial statement and do a budget and track our spending. These things are natural to me, so I do think that helps me right now."

One of the key challenges Kwajelyn has faced with all the back-and-forth since *Roe* was overturned has been keeping staff morale up. When we first talked with Kwajelyn several months before *Dobbs*, she told us that morale had already been low going into the year because of the pandemic. On top of that, she was beginning to have conversations with staff about what a future without *Roe* would mean. She told us that she was being "honest and realistic about the threat that is coming." She told her staff that "abortion is on the chopping block and there is a very real possibility that we won't be able to provide it at some point. Until then, let's figure out what we need to do to make sure that everybody who is getting abortions today can get them."

In the midst of July, after *Dobbs*, when the clinic doubled its patient volume, Kwajelyn paid close attention to her staff's well-being. Most were doing OK, but the phone center staff was slammed with calls from all over the South. Increasing the challenge for her staff in the month after *Dobbs*, antiabortion extremists invaded Feminist Women's. "It was three individuals," Kwajelyn told us, "and they were let in because it was a wellness day and people behind the desk assumed they had an appointment. They mostly just came in and prayed and screamed and videotaped around the waiting room before they were escorted out." Kwajelyn was most concerned that her staff should feel protected. She acknowledged that this type of violence as well as everyday harassment and political attacks make abortion provision "dangerous. It's as secure as a cracker. It feels very fragile for people."

Thankfully, as a result of her financial planning and creativity, Kwajelyn has been able not only to avoid layoffs but also to give her staff a well-deserved pay increase since *Dobbs*. Especially amidst the post-*Dobbs* chaos, Kwajelyn said she felt "a tremendous responsibility for everybody on staff, for making sure that folks are OK." So she worked to make sure that her staff in this particularly difficult year earned not just a living wage but a "thriving wage," as she called it. With the mindset that she is "walking in an abundance posture as opposed to a scarcity posture," she was able to work the budget to provide a staggered cost-of-living adjustment that decreased the gap between the highest- and lowest-paid staff.

Kwajelyn felt at the end of the year that this was the right thing to do to acknowledge "the exhaustion and the overwhelm with trying to make sure that the staff clearly understand everything that's happening at any given moment in a way that they can explain to patients. I think that's just really tiring." Six months after *Dobbs*, she was proud that there had not been a lot of turnover beyond the usual. "I think a lot of folks here continue to be really dedicated and committed to their work and the importance of our work."

AN IMMEDIATE TRIGGER

On the other side of the country, in Utah, Karrie Galloway experienced her own whiplash after *Dobbs*. Karrie had been working at Planned Parenthood Association of Utah for over forty years, and as the executive director for over thirty-five of those years, when we first talked with her in 2022. She saw the writing on the wall well before the *Dobbs* decision: "I stuck with this job because it never got boring. Now it's a little more exciting than I need in my life. I could go with boring." Boring is not what she got. Instead, like in the clichéd action movie with the police officer catching a career-defining case right before retiring, Karrie experienced everything that overturning *Roe* could throw at her the year before she retired.

Karrie grew up in Wisconsin as a "gal of the sixties," in her words. Her family was "very Catholic": her grandmother used to tell Karrie that her mother "would go to hell because she practiced contraception." But that didn't sit right for Karrie, who knew that her parents were good people who "brought us up that you had to give back to the community." Her parents' message and life made her a believer in the importance of the availability of contraception and of doing good from an early age.

In college Karrie saw her commitment broaden. She went to Planned Parenthood for her own care, believed in women's health and good sex, and volunteered as a model patient at the university medical school so doctors could learn how to do Pap smears from someone "telling them what they were doing right and wrong." She graduated with a degree in teaching and, after teaching at the university, moved to Utah. The attraction was the state's outdoor recreation—backpacking, skiing, river-running.

Once in Utah, she and her husband began thinking about having kids, a decision that brought her to Planned Parenthood. As she related to us, the discussion with her husband was "Should we have our own kids? Was that selfish? Should we co-parent? Should we adopt? So we took a class from Planned Parenthood in options in pregnancy." That class exposed her to a job opening in Planned Parenthood's education department.

Karrie applied for the position, got it, and never looked back. Hired in 1981, her teaching degree made her a natural fit for the education department. From there, she became the manager of the department; then the assistant director who managed the clinics for the Utah affiliate; then, in 1987, the chief executive officer of the entire affiliate. She held that position until early 2023, when she retired, a couple of months after our last interview with her.

When we first talked with Karrie about her expectations for the year, she was optimistic about her affiliate's opportunity to survive. The "small but mighty" affiliate had eight clinics, three of them providing abortion. Two of those provide only medication abortion and one, the Salt Lake City center, offers procedural abortions as well. Karrie stressed that everything she told us should be attributed to the team of people at the affiliate and its supporters, not just to her. "I acknowledge I am the leader and the storyteller," she said, "but it was all of us who made it work. In reality, there's not much I do alone without consulting with the team."

Karrie was very proud of all that her team has been able to accomplish in Utah. "We have always been innovative, kind of a little cowboyish in doing it ourselves," and she insisted that those who fight for reproductive autonomy in a state like Utah are possibly stronger than they are elsewhere because they have to "gather tightly together to show their resistance and their strength." Amid some difficult times in the state, the affiliate has "figured out how to make it work," in part because they have been successful in "finding friends who helped us interpret the law."

This description turned out to be prescient for what happened throughout the rest of 2022, which was marked by many of the same legal twists and turns that Kwajelyn faced in Georgia. One of the biggest battles Karrie faced came in the hours and days immediately after *Dobbs* was decided.

Utah, like many states, had a trigger law banning abortion at any stage of pregnancy with only limited exceptions for rape, incest, and risk to the life of the person who is pregnant or to a major bodily function.[6] The law was passed in 2020 when the legislators knew that it was unconstitutional because of *Roe v. Wade*, so they wrote a trigger into the law in the form of a contingent effective date. That provision stated that the law would not take effect until the legislature's general counsel certifies that a state or federal appellate court has ruled that states can ban abortion. In other words, the law would take effect when *Roe* was overruled.

When we talked with Karrie before *Dobbs* was decided, she had been optimistic that the trigger law would not kick in immediately upon any Supreme Court decision overturning *Roe*. In preparation for the Court's decision, Planned Parenthood had talked with the legislative office responsible for the trigger implementation and had asked if they could have a few days before the trigger is pulled. Planned Parenthood argued that there was some ambiguity about the law's exceptions and the rules regulating how the trigger would work. Karrie acknowledged that this request was "hopeful thinking" but nonetheless tried to push government officials to confirm this buffer period. No matter what happened with *Dobbs*, though, Karrie was adamant that, because Planned Parenthood provides other care besides abortion in Utah, "Our doors stay open. Damn straight they do."

Karrie's hopeful thinking was not borne out by reality. Less than twelve hours after *Dobbs* was decided, the Utah trigger ban took effect. For Karrie, the whiplash was real. She learned that the law had taken effect the Friday evening of the decision, right before the start of a big protest rally. Karrie and her colleagues had cared for patients all day after *Dobbs* was decided. Together with various community groups they had planned to hold a march when the decision was announced, so on that Friday night, the community showed up to "process what happened." At the event many people from all different communities in the area spoke movingly about their abortion stories or their commitment to abortion as a right.

The event lasted until 9 p.m., when Karrie and her team had to start planning how to care for patients now that abortion was illegal in Utah. Their highest priority was determining what to do for two patients who were in the midst of a two-day procedure known as dilation and evacuation. Most in-clinic first-trimester abortions, whether procedural or with medication, involve a clinic visit of just a few hours, but for patients later in pregnancy the procedure can take two days—on day one the patient's body is prepared and on day two the patient returns to the clinic to complete the abortion.

Karrie's clinic had two patients who had their day one appointment on the Friday *Dobbs* was decided, which meant they had to return to complete the procedure on Saturday. However, Friday night Utah's trigger law had kicked in, meaning abortion was now illegal in the state. Did that now mean that the patients could not get care the next day?

To Karrie and the doctors who worked at her clinic, despite the legal back-and-forth, what they should do was clear: "We have to complete it. Because otherwise the woman would be in jeopardy. On Saturday we had to complete that procedure." She and her colleagues made sure to "document the hell out of that procedure so it was clear that it had to be done." With this precaution as well as consulting with their lawyers, the doctors and Karrie were comfortable that what they were doing was within the bounds of law and consistent with the proper practice of medicine.

Unfortunately, though, Karrie and her colleagues had to turn away the other patients who came to the clinic Saturday morning. As she put it, starkly, "All other people had to be told that they no longer had bodily autonomy." What particularly troubled Karrie was that the women she turned away that day had already rearranged their lives to get their abortion. Utah had a law that required people seeking an abortion to consent to the abortion first and then wait at least seventy-two hours before getting the abortion. The people who were on the schedule for Saturday had already gone through the consent process and had planned their schedule and lives around having an abortion that day. "These people's lives were thrown for a loop. They had gone through all the steps and done everything the state told them they had to do to get this procedure." But because the legislative counsel certified the trigger ban Friday night, "they lost their bodily autonomy on Saturday."

The clinic was open that weekend, but on Monday the only option Karrie and her team had was to refer patients to other providers. They would have liked to be able to do a "warm" referral, where the staff connects patients to providers directly and helps them make their appointments. However, Karrie decided that under Utah law it was now too risky to be involved in connecting the patient to the provider because it may be seen as aiding someone in violating the law. The only safe option left to her staff was to refer patients to a website that they would have to use on their own to find the closest abortion provider in another state. These two days of being able to do nothing more than "sending people out in the cold" were some of the hardest days for Karrie and her staff.

Despite the ban being in effect, on Monday morning, three days after *Dobbs*, women seeking an abortion had shown up at the clinic hoping that the law might change. They had good reason to be hopeful. Karrie's lawyers had been planning for this moment and filed a complaint on Planned Parenthood's behalf for immediate injunctive relief from a state court once the trigger law went into effect. The court held a virtual hearing at 3 p.m. on Monday, and the judge ruled immediately that the state ban would be put on hold until further proceedings in two weeks.

The patience and foresight of the women in the clinic waiting room paid off. The moment Karrie heard the judge announce that the law was blocked, she went downstairs to tell them the good news: "He just granted the order. We have to wait until he signs it, but you guys can get ready to start providing care." Her staff all cheered. To the women waiting she said, "It's your lucky day. We're going to see you today." Having waited all day on the hope that the judge would grant the injunction, they were all incredibly relieved. Karrie's staff also reached out to everyone who had come in on Saturday or who had left earlier in the day and told them they could now come back if they wanted.

The order prevented the law from going into effect only for two weeks, at which point the judge would have to decide whether to grant an injunction putting the law on hold for the entire length of the litigation. Despite the possibility that Karrie, her staff, and her patients might be right back in the same situation two weeks later, Karrie said that Monday, when the trigger law was first blocked, was a day of celebration after the whiplash of the weekend.

Karrie and her staff celebrated again two weeks later when the judge issued a preliminary injunction putting the law on hold for the entirety of the litigation. He reasoned that people in Utah would face "irreparable harm" and there would be "increased health risks" if he didn't issue the injunction. A month later the Utah attorney general appealed this ruling to the state supreme court, and in October, the Utah Supreme Court ruled that it would hear the appeal but that the injunction would remain in force until final decision. As of June 2024 the court had not yet ruled.

While this legal wrangling played out, Karrie and her clinic provided lawful, safe abortions for the rest of the year. When we talked with her at the end of 2022, she told us that since the initial weekend after *Roe* was overturned and the clinic briefly had to cease providing care, Karrie and her staff had performed about a thousand abortions for patients seeking their services.

Even though abortion had been legal in Utah for that entire time, Karrie and her staff had to wage other legal battles. The same day that Planned Parenthood got its first injunction blocking the trigger ban, another state abortion restriction took effect. In 2019 Utah had banned abortions starting at eighteen weeks of pregnancy. This law never took effect while *Roe* was the law of the land because a federal court issued an injunction putting it on hold. However, once *Roe* was overturned, the state went back to the federal court and asked it to lift the injunction. That happened on the Monday after *Dobbs*. So at almost the same moment the trigger ban was blocked, the eighteen-week ban took effect. Karrie described this back-and-forth with the state as a "checkmate match. Except they're using people's lives in the game."

"PERSONHOOD"

And then there are the unanswered legal questions. Much has been made of these uncertainties since *Roe* was overruled, especially when it comes to care for people later in pregnancy facing medical emergencies. The ultimately unsuccessful state lawsuit in Texas discussed in the introductory chapter attempted to clarify some of these issues. There, a state court was asked to explain how the state's abortion ban's exceptions work. The problem is that both in Texas and elsewhere it's unclear what exactly constitutes a threat to the patient's life under the exception. Without clarity, doctors are often too scared to provide care for their patients because if they make a mistake, they risk going to jail for life if a jury later believes there was no emergency. As a result, patients are struggling to get care for emergencies that arise during pregnancy. The Texas Supreme Court was unmoved by this argument, so the confusion remains.[7]

This has been a familiar part of the post-*Roe* landscape, with horror stories appearing in the news almost daily. Many abortion advocates view maintaining this uncertainty as an intentional tactic. The law appears more politically reasonable than a complete ban because it has an exception for the pregnant woman's safety, but because doctors are too scared of the consequences of making a mistake, very few are comfortable using it. Consequently almost no abortions take place under the emergency provision. This is a win-win for abortion opponents: they look more reasonable in the public eye, but in reality no abortions are being performed.

Both Kwajelyn and Karrie spent the months after *Dobbs* dealing with legal uncertainties of their own. In Georgia, Kwajelyn faced a novel "personhood" law that the Georgia legislature had passed in 2019.[8] The Georgia legislature declared that a fertilized egg is a legal person for all purposes under Georgia law. This provision is contained in the same law that banned abortions after six weeks of pregnancy. When a federal court blocked the six-week ban from taking effect in 2019, it also blocked the personhood provisions. After *Dobbs*, when the federal appeals court lifted the injunction for the six-week ban, it also lifted the injunction for the personhood provision in the law.

So what does this mean now? In July 2022, an Arizona federal judge blocked that state's personhood law, saying that it is "anyone's guess" what the law would mean. An abortion provider could be following the state's abortion laws—performing an abortion that complied with the specific provisions governing abortion—but, because of the personhood law, might be guilty of murder because the state now considers the fetus a person. Because of this problem, the Arizona federal judge ruled that the statute was unconstitutionally vague, writing, "Medical providers should not have to guess about whether the otherwise lawful performance of their jobs could lead to criminal, civil, or professional liability."[9]

In Georgia, however, the personhood law sprang back into effect, leaving Kwajelyn and her colleagues trying to figure out what it meant. When we talked with her before *Dobbs*, she expressed some concern about this uncertainty, telling us that the state had assured the public that the personhood provision does not ban abortions before six weeks. Even so she worried that local prosecutors could decide that in their view the fetus is a person, so even under six weeks an abortion would be manslaughter or homicide. Because of the state's assurances, Kwajelyn wasn't overly concerned, but she acknowledged that there was "a little bit of risk involved" because of the uncertainty as to how the law could be interpreted.

After *Roe* was overturned, Kwajelyn maintained the same position, saying that the clinic would continue to operate based on the assurances the state had given the public that abortion remains legal through six weeks "until we learn otherwise." She recognized that "the risk still exists theoretically," but was comfortable taking that risk. One of the factors adding to her comfort level was the fact that several Georgia district attorneys, including the DA covering Atlanta, where Feminist Women's is located, had spoken out saying that they are going to use their prosecutorial discretion not to prosecute abortion cases within their jurisdiction. "Maybe I'm being naïve at this point," Kwajelyn said, "but I think some of this stuff is a lot of talk. Because they are really counting on that chilling effect. They really want us to be scared to move. But I don't think they actually want to act in some of these cases. That's what it feels like so far."

ABORTION PILLS

Because of the uncertainty around Georgia's personhood law, Kwajelyn and her clinic have been more cautious about treating patients traveling from other parts of the state who opt for a medication abortion. The normal protocol for a medication abortion is for a patient to take the first drug, mifepristone, at the health center, which causes the pregnancy to stop developing, and then four pills of the second medication, misoprostol, which causes the uterus to contract and expel the pregnancy, at home. Because of Georgia's personhood law, Kwajelyn's clinic encourages travelers to take all of the pills in a county with a friendly prosecutor before they return home to a county with a potentially less-friendly prosecutor. Especially if there are complications that lead to the patient's seeking follow-up care at a hospital, Kwajelyn would prefer for that to happen "where the likelihood of them being investigated or scrutinized is lower because of the potential for the patient being criminalized under the personhood provision."

Karrie faced similar challenges in Utah. If the patient returns home to a state with an abortion ban and takes the second set of pills there, Karrie expressed uncertainty as to whether the clinic or the patient would face legal trouble. She told us before *Dobbs* that this problem was foremost on her mind for patients who travel from Idaho into Utah to get abortion pills.

Once the Supreme Court allowed states to ban abortion and Idaho did so, Karrie instituted a policy that some other clinics have adopted, one that proved controversial. The Planned Parenthood health center in Utah that is closest to the Idaho border provides only medication abortion. Because of Idaho's ban and the risk of an antiabortion prosecutor there, the affiliate told patients coming to Utah from Idaho that they have to travel further and go to Salt Lake City to get a procedural abortion. Without the ability to force Idaho residents to stay in Utah long enough to take all of the pills involved in a medication abortion, Karrie said that the potential legal liability was just too problematic for her providers. She recognizes that this extra travel requirement poses a challenge for patients and lamented that the affiliate made this decision, but, she said, "We had to do it to protect our staff."

Uncertainty around medication abortion posed another challenge for Karrie. The lawsuit over mifepristone's approval that the Supreme Court ultimately dismissed in June 2024 was originally filed in late 2022. It was assigned to a conservative antiabortion federal judge, sending shockwaves through the world of abortion provision.

Because of the lawsuit, abortion providers began planning for the uncertain future. At the end of 2022, Karrie listed for us several unanswered questions raised by the case, using "mife" as shorthand for mifepristone and "miso" as shorthand for misoprostol. "What if we run out of mife? Is there enough mife in the world to stockpile? Should we be buying miso and stockpiling it? And then there's the question if we've got mife and we stockpiled it, can we still use it?" In the end Karrie expressed frustration about the uncertainty the lawsuit caused: "For administrators, it's just another goddamn thing you're dealing with."

Yet another legal unknown arose for Karrie after *Dobbs*. In September of 2022, even though the trigger ban injunction was in place, a group of antiabortion state legislators sent a cease-and-desist letter to Planned Parenthood, arguing that Karrie's affiliate, by mailing abortion pills to patients was violating a 150-year-old federal law, the Comstock Act, which prohibits, among other things, sending anything that can "produc[e] abortion" through the mail or a private express service.[10] This law, whose provisions as they relate to abortion hadn't been enforced for almost a century, is widely considered antiquated and unenforceable. However, some in the antiabortion movement have begun arguing that it should be enforced now that *Roe* has been overturned. The letter also said that if the Utah Supreme Court reverses the trigger ban injunction, then Planned Parenthood's providers will be criminally liable for all of the abortions they performed when the injunction was in place. To be clear, this is a fringe legal theory developed by one of the most extreme antiabortion legal strategists, but Karrie needed to take the threat to her staff seriously.[11]

Even though she knew the letter was "obviously a stunt," Karrie hired a criminal attorney, who discussed the risks involved with each of the affiliate's providers and their partners. Even if these two theories are unlikely to be successful, Karrie explained that "there's a lot of concern about our providers losing their license, their livelihoods, their family. That really made people nervous." Karrie and the lawyer tried to assure the affiliate's providers that the injunction did in fact protect them. They all continued to care for patients, but, Karrie said, it's all just "chaotic. Everyone is extremely stressed."

Karrie's response: Twice in the latter half of 2022 she shut the health centers for the day to have an all-staff gathering. The affiliate had never done this before, but in 2022, it felt necessary to keep the staff from being too overwhelmed with the back-and-forth and the legal uncertainty. She lamented that, while it was important to do, it wasn't enough in this chaotic year. "We're trying to ease some of the pain that we can, but there's only so much we can do because we have to provide care. We have to be in the clinic because people need care." The ultimate challenge is that a court could at any time set aside the injunction, which creates a huge degree of uncertainty. "Everyone's on edge, and there's just nothing to do to relieve that pressure."

ANTICIPATING FUTURE BANS

Even in states that had uninterrupted access in 2022, legal uncertainty caused by the overturning of *Roe* still plagued some providers because of the possibility of bans in the future. Kelly Flynn experienced this in both states where she owns and operates abortion clinics—one in Florida and three in North Carolina. With abortion banned in many of the neighboring Southern states, patients traveled from near and far to get care, and Kelly saw a huge influx of patients at all of her clinics in 2022.

When we talked with her at the end of 2022, Kelly felt terrible for patients who were struggling to figure out how to get care in this new environment. She told us, "It's so hard for me to even understand, after decades doing this, not being able to have that option. People now know it for the first time. It's just—it's unbelievable, really." Kelly's incredulousness is rooted in her own story of coming to own and operate her four clinics. Her involvement started in the 1990s, when she was a teenager and in college in North Carolina. After dating her boyfriend for about six months, she found out she was pregnant. "I was, like, pregnant? I don't want to be pregnant! What do I do?"

Kelly did what many people do. She called a friend who had previously told her about her own abortion, and that friend told her about a nearby abortion clinic. Kelly went there, had her abortion, and got her first pack of birth control pills. Being a college student who was waiting tables to make ends meet, she didn't have the money to fill a prescription on her own, so she was grateful that the clinic helped her out.

Three months later she was back at the clinic, pregnant again. "I was that person that said, it's not going to happen again. Well, it happened again, literally within the same semester." When she went back to the clinic, she found herself helping out another patient who was really scared about the procedure. Having gone through it before, Kelly knew what to expect and eased the patient's fears. "I said, you're going to be fine. So I had my procedure done. She had hers, and we wound up in the recovery room together."

And then something happened that put Kelly on the path she has been on ever since. A member of the clinic staff asked Kelly whether she wanted a job. "Literally while I was getting my abortion, they were like, 'Can you work Saturdays?'" Two weeks later, Kelly started working at the clinic, and she has been there ever since.

The clinic where she got her abortion and her first job was one of five clinics owned by the same person. Within a year Kelly was a senior manager at the clinic where she worked. Within another three years, she was a vice president of the ownership entity of all five clinics in North Carolina and Florida. The next year, because the entity underwent restructuring, she moved to Florida to work at the Jacksonville clinic, which had been affiliated with the North Carolina clinics.

Then another surprise came. Once Kelly was in Florida, the clinic owner asked her, "Do you want to buy the clinic?" Kelly thought, "'With what? You don't pay me that well!' But we figured it out, called around, I got a loan, and I bought the clinic from him when I was twenty-five." Within six years of getting her first abortion, Kelly now owned and ran an abortion clinic. As the years progressed, she expanded, buying three clinics in North Carolina—in Raleigh, Greensboro, and Charlotte. She knows this work isn't for everyone, but she said, "I don't know anything else," and she feels successful because she is doing what she loves and is meant to do.

Even though she loves her work, 2022 was hard for Kelly. Both of the states where she operates clinics changed their abortion laws because of *Dobbs*. Florida had passed a ban on abortions at fifteen weeks in the spring of 2022. The law was scheduled to take effect July 1, a week after the Supreme Court overturned *Roe*. Along with several other clinics in the state, Kelly sued in state court to block the law under the state constitution. The lawsuit met with initial success when a state court trial judge ruled that the law was likely unconstitutional and put the law on hold. His ruling took effect the morning of July 5, but later that day the state appealed, which meant, under Florida law, the fifteen-week ban automatically went back into effect.

With the constitutionality of the fifteen-week ban bouncing around, Kelly and her clinic played it cautiously and did not begin to see patients beyond fifteen weeks. They were, in her words, "too afraid" that they would start a procedure and then in the middle of the day the courts would reinstate the law and the clinic would be caught in a bind. So after the law went into effect on July 1, Kelly's clinic did not see patients beyond fifteen weeks.

The change from providing abortions through twenty-four weeks to stopping at fifteen weeks was significant for Kelly's clinic. It had previously been the only full-time second-trimester abortion provider in northern Florida, so this was a big adjustment. However, patients adapted better than Kelly had anticipated. The clinic's numbers dropped a bit, but more patients came in for earlier abortions than before. Kelly attributed this to a combination of greater awareness about the need to get to clinics earlier in pregnancy as well as increased resources for patients. Because the abortion rights movement had seen an increase in funding to help patients access abortion by assisting them in getting to clinics (discussed in greater depth in chapter 7), patients who had previously delayed getting their abortion because they were having trouble finding money to pay for it or traveling to a clinic were having fewer problems. She told us that now, "if they call and say, 'I'm at the point I just found out I am pregnant, but I'm short this much money,' we've got them covered. We've got transportation covered, we've got hotel costs covered, so that seems to be driving more patients to be seen before fifteen weeks."

Florida's gestational limit remained at fifteen weeks for the rest of 2022, but Kelly still faced much uncertainty as the calendar flipped to 2023. When we talked to her at the end of 2022, Governor Ron DeSantis had just won reelection, so everyone in the state was waiting to see whether he and the legislature would push for even more abortion restrictions. She told us, "I'm nervous. My understanding is they have a special session coming up and are entertaining a full ban or the six-week ban. It's hard to tell with him because he's so unpredictable."

What Kelly feared at the end of 2022 materialized in 2023 when the Florida legislature enacted a six-week ban that included a provision that it would take effect only after the state supreme court ruled on the already existing fifteen-week ban. The court took its time with that case, but eventually, in April 2024, the court found the fifteen-week ban constitutional, thus paving the way for the six-week ban to take effect on May 1. As of mid-2024, Florida has become a state with seriously limited abortion access. Compounding the back-and-forth, it's very possible that may change as a result of the outcome of a ballot initiative in November 2024 that would enshrine the right to abortion in the state constitution.[12]

Abortion's uncertain future in Florida at the end of 2022 impacted Kelly in one other important way. In early 2022 she had told us about her plans to open a new clinic in the Florida Panhandle. She had just purchased a building that she was hoping to convert to an abortion clinic by the end of the year. The building had other medical tenants, but their leases were supposed to end over the course of the year, at which point the abortion clinic would open. She did this because of the abortion bans she saw coming in other Southern states, and it would be much easier for patients coming from Mississippi, Alabama, Louisiana, and maybe even Tennessee to get to the western part of the Panhandle than to Jacksonville, which is on the Atlantic coast in the eastern part of the state.

As of the end of 2022 the new clinic was still on hold. One of the previous tenants was still in the property, so Kelly was still waiting for her to move out. After that Kelly would need to jump through a few more administrative hoops, which was expected to take about three months, and then she could open. But with the political uncertainty in the state about a possible stricter abortion ban on the horizon, she was not disappointed things hadn't moved more quickly.

"In some sense," she explained, "I'm not opening the Panhandle clinic until we know what the law looks like." She mused that the uncertainty over Florida's abortion future was "kind of a blessing in disguise. Because, I think that, had the property already been available, I would've already invested and opened a clinic there."

Since things had taken longer than she expected, she hoped to have more complete knowledge about the legal landscape before opening the Panhandle clinic. At the end of 2022, we asked her if she would still open in the Panhandle if the state enacted a six-week ban, and she replied, "Yeah, I would still try. I'm not going to close. I'm going to try to accommodate everybody and anybody that we can. If there's a six-week ban, then we just go with it and we figure it out." But as of mid-2024 the clinic was still not open.

In North Carolina, Kelly faces a different situation. In that state, her three clinics did not immediately have to change their level of care because of *Dobbs*. They had previously performed abortions only up to twenty weeks of pregnancy in the state, the same gestational limit that became state law after *Roe* was overturned.

The uncertainty in the state came from North Carolina having a pro-choice governor with an antiabortion legislature. Kelly told us before *Dobbs* that she hoped North Carolina would "be safe for a while now," but she was trying not to get her "hopes up to be set up for disappointment." Kelly worried that the legislature might override any veto from Governor Roy Cooper.

The worries she had in 2022 came to pass in 2023. The North Carolina legislature passed a ban on abortion at twelve weeks. Governor Cooper did veto it, but one Democratic state legislator flipped parties and voted with the antiabortion Republican bloc, so the legislature was able to override the governor's veto. Kelly's North Carolina clinics, like all of the other clinics in the state, had to pivot to stop delivering second-trimester care once the twelve-week ban went into effect in July 2023.[13]

These setbacks didn't stop Kelly from looking for ways to continue to serve patients in the South. In early 2024, she opened a new clinic in Danville, Virginia, just over the border from North Carolina.[14] The new clinic expands service in a state that most think will see travelers from Florida and North Carolina now that, post-*Dobbs*, they have lowered their gestational age limits.

CONFUSION

Providing abortion care in 2022 in states like those where Kwajelyn, Karrie, and Kelly work was not easy. The whiplash. The chaos. The confusion. With *Roe*, there was some lack of clarity about how state restrictions worked, but there was always the baseline rule that abortion had to be legal until viability.

With *Dobbs*, that baseline is gone. As Kelly summed it up for us, the situation "confuses so many people, staff included. Just to go back and forth on it. It's so unfair. It's unfair to the medical community. It's unfair to the patients."

CHAPTER FIVE

SURGE STATES

*We anticipated a higher call volume, but we
didn't anticipate a four times higher call volume
in the first several days after Dobbs.*

—ERIN KING, Hope Clinic

The impact of *Dobbs* wasn't just clinic closures, provider creativity, and managing chaos. Clinics in states where abortion remained legal, and especially those that were closer to states where abortion became illegal, saw a huge influx in patients. In late 2023, the Guttmacher Institute released data comparing abortion numbers in various states in 2020 to those in the first six months of 2023. In Colorado the number of abortions increased by 89 percent; in Illinois, by 69 percent; in New Mexico, by 220 percent; in Washington State, by 36 percent; and in California by 16 percent.[1]

In this chapter we highlight the experiences of people working in leadership positions in clinics from these five "surge" states who worked mightily in the face of many challenges to serve their patients in the face of the increase in volume in response to the crisis of *Dobbs*. Colorado, New Mexico, and Illinois have been some of the best-positioned states to meet the needs of abortion seekers in nearby states. Located in or near the middle of the country and bordering large states with abortion bans, these three states saw an influx that required clinics there to open new facilities, experiment with new delivery models, and accommodate travelers in ways they never had to before.

Location meant something else to states that were further from population-rich states with abortion bans. In those states, such as California and Washington, where abortion remained legal, providers were not hit as hard. Nevertheless, even a modest increase in patients meant clinics in those states had to adapt their services in various ways to the new environment.

The leaders covered in this chapter highlight the complexity of working in a surge state at a time when almost twenty states ban or severely restrict abortion. On the one hand, through the almost-miraculous efforts of the people profiled in this chapter, their colleagues, and many others like them, clinics in surge states have met the moment and been able to make the necessary changes and sacrifices to care for the patients who have flocked to see them from all over the country. On the other hand, their experiences make very clear that caring for this many patients presents monumental challenges, chief among them obtaining and sustaining necessary staffing levels, attending to staff morale, and dealing with the logistics of having so many out-of-town patients. Whether the efforts detailed here are sustainable in the long run is still unknown.

COLORADO AND NEW MEXICO

Because of SB8 in Texas, Planned Parenthood of the Rocky Mountains (PPRM), the Planned Parenthood affiliate based in Denver that covers Colorado, New Mexico, Wyoming, and southern Nevada, had been experiencing a huge upsurge of patients since late 2021. The struggles of many of these patients traveling from Texas prefigured the situations that would become commonplace after *Dobbs*.

Vicki Cowart, the outgoing long-standing CEO of PPRM, recounted to us one particularly memorable incident that revealed the desperation of traveling patients determined to get an abortion, no matter the obstacles. The patient had driven twelve hours from Texas to Colorado in a snowstorm. Her mother apparently had been admitted to an Alzheimer's unit the previous day, and her daughter was uneasy about leaving her, so she took her mother with her. "She had her mother and her mother's caregiver in the car with her," Vicki told us. "And the patient was just like, 'I got to take care of this woman and I got to have an abortion, all in the same day.'"

The absurdity of the situation, as Vicki made clear, was that this twenty-four-hour round-trip drive (not counting the time in the health center) was to receive pills for a medication abortion—pills that, in a rational world, she would have obtained locally or received in the mail. Vicki told us in disbelief, "I think this just so encapsulates what women are going though. And bear in mind, this woman had the wherewithal. She had a car that worked.

She had money for gas. She had a caretaker for her mother. Imagine if any of those things had not been true."

When we talked with Vicki in early 2022, she was in the process of handing off the affiliate leadership to Adrienne Mansanares. Vicki had been CEO for almost two decades and had been mentoring Adrienne to fill her shoes for years before we talked with them. Adrienne came to this work because of her long love for Planned Parenthood. She recounted to us how her "very big Hispanic family" had been in southern Colorado for generations. Growing up, she moved around, from Colorado to New Mexico to Nevada and back. "My family loves family," she said, but she grew up not sure that she wanted children herself. Now she is married and has two children, five years apart; her pregnancies were planned. She owes that to the years of reduced-cost birth control she received from Planned Parenthood. In fact, she said, "I'm where I am today because of Planned Parenthood." And when we asked her specifically why she said that, she responded, "It's birth control, birth control, birth control."

Adrienne didn't start her career at Planned Parenthood. She had been working for a community foundation doing community organization and racial equity work when a friend who was a board member at PPRM approached her about joining the board. Adrienne, almost thirty at the time, joined and eventually became the board's chair. In that role, she was very active with the organization but in a volunteer role. Soon, however, Vicki started looking toward her eventual retirement, and she approached Adrienne as a likely successor as CEO. After consulting with her family about the sacrifices inherent in the role with time away from family, along with safety and security issues, Adrienne said yes.

As she began her new role as CEO in early 2022, Adrienne was bracing herself for an increased workload in a system already strained by SB8. Before SB8, the Guttmacher Institute reported, an average of more than 4,800 legal abortions a month took place in Texas.[2] To be clear, not all Texans needing abortions under SB8 or the post-*Dobbs* ban went to Colorado and New Mexico, but the huge influx of Texans fleeing for care into Colorado and New Mexico because of SB8 was undoubtedly going to increase once *Roe* fell. And with *Dobbs* allowing other states to ban abortion as well, that number was going to be even higher once people started traveling to Colorado and New Mexico from everywhere.

Also challenging for PPRM at this time, like all healthcare entities, were lingering issues resulting from the Covid-19 pandemic. Supply chain difficulties and, above all, recruiting and retaining of staff across the larger healthcare labor market were the most significant of these challenges. Though Adrienne and her leadership team were eager to expand the organization's offerings, both by opening new health centers and adding access and capacity to existent ones, such an expansion was difficult. Speaking of her postponed wish to add a new procedure room in one of her main health centers in Colorado, she exclaimed, "I've waited for two months to get a new exam table!"

The labor shortages associated with the pandemic posed a separate challenge in preparing for *Dobbs* as they delayed the construction of new facilities. PPRM had to deal with a shortage of contractors during that period, a problem many organizations faced. But this problem was compounded for Planned Parenthood: even contractors with no ideological objections to abortion often hesitate to work with Planned Parenthood because of fears of antiabortion vandalism at the worksite or of being boycotted by others. Adrienne told us that PPRM had been planning a new health center in Albuquerque for three years, but that construction had been delayed because of labor issues, a consequence of both limited contractor availability and the stigma attached to Planned Parenthood in some quarters. The security concerns around this facility, which opened and began seeing patients in December 2023, were such that Adrienne told a reporter that she herself was not privy to the actual location of the new building before it opened.[3]

Anticipating how the Supreme Court would rule, Adrienne was still determined to expand the affiliate to meet the need of Texans and people traveling from other states. Among many other initiatives, she set into motion plans for a new health center. Adrienne stressed, "We're not going to go into a community that has not known us or seen us." Fortunately, PPRM had spent years establishing relationships with reproductive justice organizations in southern New Mexico. Adrienne told us that these community leaders expressed enthusiastic support for a facility in Las Cruces, New Mexico's second-largest city.

Las Cruces is very close to the Texas border and, as Adrienne explained to us, is also a healthcare desert, lacking medical facilities for local New Mexicans who are in serious need of sexual and reproductive healthcare of all kinds. In explaining the process of establishing this new health center to us, Adrienne stressed that it was important that she had met with local FBI agents to ascertain the climate of the area with respect to safety for an abortion clinic. PPRM's new Las Cruces health center eventually opened in May 2023.

When *Dobbs* hit, a surge of patients traveled to PPRM for care. Adrienne noted the heightened stress among abortion-care patients who had to travel to Colorado or New Mexico. Contrasting the post-*Dobbs* situation with the situation before *Dobbs* and SB8, she said, "Everybody who's coming from Texas has a story, and it's not a good story. We're not in the phase of, 'Oh, abortion is a safe and simple procedure' anymore.' No, it's not. It's instead this cataclysmic thing in your life where you have to figure out how to get time off from work and find the money and get someone to take care of your kids."

Not surprisingly, the reality that so many abortion care patients suddenly had to travel meant that their need for financial and logistical assistance increased dramatically after SB8 and *Dobbs*. As discussed in further detail in chapter 7, local and national abortion funds have played a central role in enabling abortion care post-*Dobbs*, and this was true for PPRM as well. Drawing on funds raised by loyal local donors from a range of economic backgrounds as well as national organizations such as the Planned Parenthood Federation of America and the National Abortion Federation, PPRM was able to allocate a considerable amount of money and staff time to help out-of-state patients. Before *Dobbs*, Adrienne said, the organization was spending about $10,000 per month on financial support for travel; in July 2022, the first month after *Dobbs*, the figure climbed to $60,000. PPRM doesn't subsidize only travel. Before *Dobbs*, it had spent roughly $1 million annually subsidizing abortions for the majority of its abortion patients who are low-income; since *Dobbs*, that number has reached almost $10 million.

Like many clinics elsewhere in the country, PPRM supported its patients with "patient navigators" whose job was to help with the logistics of travel and aid in locating an appointment in the PPRM network. Adrienne spoke with admiration of the work of the patient navigators and others in the organization who had adjusted to the new post-*Dobbs* realities and worked tirelessly to aid out-of-state patients, saying, "Our partnerships are so strong. Not only with abortion-care funds, but local hotel systems, the restaurants. We're figuring out different airline nuances of how to get patients on [flights]. We've had to reroute patients when there was a blizzard here in Denver, for example. So, a patient was flying in from Dallas and we had to figure out how to get her into Las Vegas. So, I would say, with the certainty that came out of the Supreme Court ruling, we're not holding our breath for anyone to come save us. It is very much like, 'All right, let's get going.' And I love it. I'm very proud of all that."

Adrienne's pride in her organization's response did not blind her to the myriad problems the organization still faced. A major one was the ultimate fate of abortion pills, in light of the lawsuit an antiabortion group brought to overturn the FDA's 2000 approval of the drug regimen, or to reimpose medically unnecessary restrictions on the availability of abortion pills.[4] The case was dismissed in June 2024, but providers like Adrienne faced uncertainty in 2022 after the case was filed because one possible outcome was that healthcare providers might not have been able to offer medication abortion via telehealth, that is, through video appointments with a patient in her home, after which she could pick up the pills at the clinic or have them mailed directly to her. Adrienne was particularly worried about this possibility because medication abortion via telehealth is a much-needed service for her patients and plays a central role in PPRM's abortion provision. The inability to provide abortion in this way would be a crushing blow, Adrienne said.

Despite these myriad problems, the principal problem PPRM faced in the immediate months after *Dobbs* remained simply meeting the demands of so many people searching for appointments. In the twelve months after *Dobbs* the number of abortions PPRM provided for out-of-state patients increased by 124 percent over the number in the twelve months before *Dobbs*. The average straight-line "as the crow flies" distance traveled by out-of-state patients to access care at PPRM in the year after *Dobbs* was a whopping 684 miles. And the clinic's telephone system was overwhelmed. Adrienne said with exasperation, "Our wait times sometimes are as high as three hours to get an appointment. . . . Three hours on hold! Who does that?"

Yet another problem PPRM faces, shared to a degree by all Planned Parenthood facilities in states where abortion remains legal, is the potential that time and resources spent on abortion care sought by out-of-state patients will jeopardize the ability to provide the non-abortion services to local patients that have traditionally been the majority of the organization's offerings. "How many STIs [sexually transmitted infections] that are asymptomatic will go undetected without a visit?" In lamenting the lost services, Adrienne said, "It's birth control, and it's cervical cancer screenings."

When the organization opens scheduling templates for patients to make appointments online, Adrienne said, "They are filling with abortion care visits. We can't then do the walk-in of someone who is like, 'I think I have an STI. Can I get a test?' So, we're having to move them to an already strained public health system where they may receive rushed or stigmatizing care. I have to keep watching the percentage of our visits that will become abortion-care visits at the expense of family planning and sexual health visits. We're not helping people plan pregnancies. We're solving what happens when we don't get to."

Indeed, by summer 2023, after we had completed our interviews with Adrienne, she candidly discussed the situation in New Mexico with a reporter, saying that demands for abortion care, mainly from Texas patients, meant both that waiting time for an abortion was then fourteen days and that other reproductive health services had to be dispersed throughout health centers in more remote areas of the state.[5] The situation in Colorado has become relatively easier as PPRM implemented a plan whereby all thirteen Planned Parenthood health centers in the state would provide medication abortion, including via telehealth where appropriate.

The patient surge at PPRM also created staffing issues. The staffing challenges that PPRM faced in 2022 were partly a function of the national labor shortages associated with the pandemic, but they were also partly a result of the new normal in abortion care in surge states that saw an explosion of patients. Even before *Dobbs*, PPRM had seen a significant increase, not only from Texas but also from Oklahoma and other states where abortion access was becoming increasingly difficult. Right before Vicki Cowart left PPRM, she had commented on the pressures this influx of patients created for the staff: "Our docs and our staff take to heart the needs of the patients so strongly. And I've tried to say to them, they're now operating in a theater of war. It's not their fault that they're not able to provide the care to all the people with extraordinary circumstances, but they still take it to heart and feel guilty about it. The mental health stress on the providers, I think, is extreme."

Fortunately, PPRM did not suffer from the shortage of doctors providing abortion care that has been a major problem in some corners of the abortion-provision world. The affiliate had a good supply of doctors before *Dobbs* and received even more inquiries from physicians in states with bans after *Dobbs*. Moreover, as Adrienne pointed out, two states in which the organization's care took place—Colorado and New Mexico—permitted advance practice clinicians, such as nurse practitioners, to provide medication abortion care.

The staffing concern that PPRM faced was in administrative support. During the Covid-19 pandemic the affiliate had faced turnover in accountants, human resources professionals, and facilities maintenance people. And, like other clinics, PPRM faced an especially acute shortage of registered nurses and medical assistants because other types of medical facilities offered higher salaries.

As a result of these intertwined problems of potential staff burnout and staff shortages, the organization made continued and conscious efforts post-*Dobbs* to invest in staff. Adrienne told us, "We strive to offer generous benefits, really recognizing that people's lives are complicated, and everyone needs to take time off as needed. We're over-hiring so that we can get people trained up, so they're not feeling alone, or like they're the only people who can provide the care. And every manager has a budget to use at their discretion for their team to build health and connection."

In our last conversation with Adrienne, she reflected on what 2022 had brought to her organization. She restated what she had said to us in an earlier interview: she and her colleagues were "hunkering down for a generation-long crisis" in the battle for reproductive rights and justice. She spoke with evident frustration of the unending presence of protesters at different PPRM sites. She was also deeply frustrated by the barrage of lawsuits or other legal maneuvers brought by abortion opponents, both nationally and regionally, which she referred to as the "weaponization of the court system." The regional actions originated in conservative areas of her largely supportive states; she spoke specifically of ordinances in small towns in both New Mexico and Colorado that antiabortion groups used to attempt to keep out new abortion facilities.

These legal clashes, she pointed out, "bleed into more hateful rhetoric and acts of violence. So, we have more threats, more threatening words that our security team catches on social media that then have to be dealt with." Like others, she drew a connection between the January 6, 2021, protesters and recent acts of violence at reproductive health centers.[6] "They're so aligned, the rhetoric, the misogynistic hateful thoughts about women." She also connected these anti-woman attacks to the ongoing attacks on transgender people and spoke with pride of the services her organization provides to transgender people.

In spite of these problems, Adrienne expressed pride at how PPRM staff at every level rose to the occasion in response to the triple challenges of Covid-19, SB8, and *Dobbs*. She also made clear to us how much she cherishes what she does. "This is the thing about this work. As soon as it really feels devastating, and I feel down, I then talk to another staff person, or I go to a health center." She was, ultimately, proud of and excited by her organization's key role in the post-*Dobbs* landscape. "Our role in the country at this historic moment is so important. And so, yes, it's heavy, but it's incredibly rewarding."

ILLINOIS

At the start of 2023, more than six months after the *Dobbs* decision, Erin King was still surprised at her deeply emotional reaction to *Dobbs*, despite all the mental preparation she had done to anticipate the outcome. An obstetrician-gynecologist and the medical director of Hope Clinic for Women in Granite City, Illinois, Erin told us that shortly after the decision was announced, she watched a movie with her clinic coworkers about the Jane Collective, a group of lay women who performed illegal abortions in Chicago in the years immediately preceding *Roe.*

Erin recalled a scene in the movie that showed a member of the collective listening to calls on an answering machine: "The women were saying, 'Please help me. Please, I need you.'" This was very emotional for Erin to watch. "I just started crying because I thought, 'Oh, my God, this is what we're living through right now.'"

The post-*Dobbs* situation was even worse than Erin had imagined it would be: "You know intellectually how bad it is, but hearing it, physically hearing how terrible it is, and how hard it is to get access, and how hard patients have worked to get to us. And these are just the patients who get to us." Speaking about the majority of her patients who now travel to her clinic, she said, "They live so far away. And a lot of our patients have never been on a plane or stayed in hotel rooms. And a fair amount of people are traveling by themselves because their support people couldn't come. And so, traveling alone to a hotel room by yourself, taking Ubers back and forth to a hotel room. It's overwhelming."

One of the many problems Erin has with this new environment is that it's not good public health. Thinking about public health has been the organizing principle of Erin's professional life. In high school and college, she focused on the small actions people can take that will have huge impacts on public health.

After considering going into adolescent medicine or contraception-based care, Erin realized abortion was the perfect answer: "Because when you do one abortion, the effect on public health, obviously, is not just one person. It's a family. It's a community. So from the aspect of looking at medicine as trying to solve one person's problem, you can fix the problem pretty quickly with an abortion. But then, also, the impacts you have on greater health. I don't think there's another answer besides abortion care." As a result, Erin has made abortion care her career. "Abortion care," she said, "there's just no greater impact that you can make day-to-day. And if there are people who are interested and passionate about it, then they should do it. And so, that's what I do."

Accordingly, Erin has been doing this work since she graduated from medical school in the early 2000s. She worked at Planned Parenthood in Chicago for a while after her residency and then moved to St. Louis for family reasons. Her Chicago associates put her in touch with the director of Hope Clinic, which hired Erin as an abortion provider. Slowly, Erin took on more responsibilities at the clinic and became the executive director in 2016, a position she held until 2023. She is now the chief medical officer at Hope Clinic while also working part-time at a federally qualified health center and delivering babies a couple times a month for a local hospital.

Hope Clinic is no stranger to out-of-town patients. Located just a short drive across the Mississippi River from St. Louis, Hope Clinic had long offered abortions to people from that city and elsewhere in Missouri, as that state became increasingly hostile to abortion care. Missouri patients had for some time made up 60 percent of the patient load. When more travelers came from Texas after the state passed SB8, the staff handled that skillfully.

Even so, anticipating the flood of patients *Dobbs* would generate caused a certain amount of panic among staff. In early 2022 Erin told us, "No matter how many times I say, 'We've been planning for this for two years and all the hiring and new equipment and scheduling has been very purposeful'—I think that they feel like there hasn't been enough planning and that this is coming and, oh, my gosh, what are we going to do, how are we going to handle this?" Their worry was that on the day of the decision "all of a sudden we will see ten thousand patients!" Erin said that she had tried to be very clear "that we are in control of our schedule and how many patients it is safe to see and all these things."

Even while staying calm, Erin knew that *Dobbs* was going to make the clinic change its practices. In the past it was able to operate with an open schedule, meaning that it would accommodate however many patients made appointments online. Now the staff was worried that "that's what's going to continue, and they'll just be here for fourteen hours a day and never go home and never eat, never sleep, and never go to the bathroom." Erin realized that the open scheduling couldn't continue. "We're all working really hard to change that mindset to us being in control of the setting. And, even though that's heartbreaking, and it means turning some patients away who need abortions, we also have to survive. We have to be functioning human beings to give good healthcare."

Unlike Planned Parenthood affiliates, Hope Clinic is a stand-alone independent abortion clinic without any national organization or big fundraising operation behind it. Erin did not have the option that many others did post-*Dobbs* to open new facilities or to change the services available at some of their satellite sites. Thus Hope Clinic's advance planning for *Dobbs* included revised budgeting scenarios for expanded staff and equipment and, of course, regular communication with lawyers about what it would mean to serve many more out-of-state patients from states with abortion bans. "We've been preparing for a couple years," Erin said. "We have an operating room that's completely outfitted, ready for patients. So there's space and there's certainly extra physician manpower, womanpower, peoplepower here, ready to go."

The flood of patients Erin had been bracing for once *Dobbs* was decided was even more overwhelming than expected. When we talked to her soon after the decision was released, Erin said, "In abortion care you're in crisis mode a lot of the time, but usually you see a light at the end of the tunnel. In this crisis, there's no tunnel, no light!" She pointed out that on June 24, the day of the decision, the "phones exploded," and as a result the types of patients who in the past could get an appointment in a few days now had to wait three weeks. "We typically get one hundred to one hundred fifty calls a day, or something like that on high-volume days," she told us. "The first couple of days we are getting six hundred calls."

This avalanche of calls, not all of which could be answered in a timely manner, led to worries about missing the most important ones. As Erin said, "When you see that there are ten calls on hold, you can't tell which of them is someone asking, 'Is abortion illegal in Illinois?' versus, 'Hi, I'm your patient and I'm bleeding.'"

Before *Dobbs*, 65 percent of Hope Clinic patients were from out of state, mainly from nearby Missouri; after *Dobbs*, that portion rose to 85 percent, and the patients came from all over the South and Midwest. This increase in traveling patients brought to the fore intertwined medical and legal issues, as well as logistical challenges. With respect to logistics, traveling patients have more difficulties arriving at the scheduled times. As Erin wryly put it, "It's really hard to say to someone, 'Oh, sorry, you're forty-five minutes late, we can't see you' when they've just driven six hours or flown three flights."

Traveling patients, Erin said, often show up more exhausted and anxious than local ones. Abortion clinics have always had patients arriving farther along in pregnancy than the patient thought she was, and this poses particular challenges when the patient is from out of town. Erin said of such situations, "So they show up, and they think they're six weeks, but they're eighteen weeks." A pregnancy this late in gestation would normally involve a more complex procedure and a longer stay in the clinic, but that is tricky to negotiate when the patient has a flight home at a fixed time.

What makes things somewhat easier facing such patient overload is the partnership that Hope Clinic forged with a Planned Parenthood clinic that opened not far away in Illinois, also close to the Missouri border. The two facilities opened a regional logistics center, with patient navigators who aid patients with arrangements for travel and lodging issues that arise. Like Adrienne, Erin marveled at the work of these patient navigators. When patients' travel plans became disrupted—for example, by a canceled or delayed flight—Erin told us that the navigators "figure it out, and suddenly the patients have a hotel room and a flight. It's like magic."

As discussed in the previous chapter, a recurring thorny issue for abortion clinics post-*Dobbs* is what protocol to use for out-of-state patients having medication abortions. Pre-*Dobbs,* the standard regimen was for the patient to take the first drug, mifepristone, at the clinic (unless the patient was in a state that allowed the drugs to be mailed to her home), and then to take the second drug, misoprostol, twenty-four or more hours later at a location of the patient's choosing, usually home.

Dobbs brought to the fore the question of when a medication abortion actually takes place. Most people in the medical profession say that taking mifepristone marks the occurrence of the abortion, as the drug causes the pregnancy tissue to stop growing. However, some lawyers have advised that hostile state prosecutors post-*Dobbs* could argue that taking misoprostol, which typically causes the expulsion of the pregnancy tissue, is the actual abortion.

As a result, many clinics in states where abortion remains legal have been wary of giving misoprostol to the patient for her to take when she returns home to a state with an abortion ban. The thinking is that taking one part of the medication abortion regimen in a state with a ban potentially puts both the patient and provider at legal risk. Because of this legal uncertainty, which remains to this day, clinics have devised different approaches to dealing with this issue. Some protected themselves by requiring patients to attest that they will stay in the clinic's state to take the second drug and complete the abortion. This protocol adds an additional cumbersome step for the patient, requiring at least one more night in a hotel, additional childcare and food expenses, another day of lost wages, and other disruptions. Hope Clinic initially adopted this protocol post-*Dobbs*, but it resulted in much patient frustration.

Under Erin's leadership, Hope Clinic changed and ultimately adopted a fairly new protocol: giving the two drugs simultaneously. This protocol had been the subject of a bulletin of the American College of Obstetricians and Gynecologists (ACOG), and information about it had been posted on the website of the National Abortion Federation (NAF)—two of the most authoritative bodies in the field of abortion provision.[7] This protocol, typically used for up to nine weeks' gestation, works well, though some patients need additional misoprostol. Both ACOG and NAF evaluated this protocol as a direct response to the issue of people traveling for medication abortion. Even so, Erin said, sighing, "Honestly, medically it's not my favorite thing to do to make a change based on what politicians think."

Erin told us that these issues related to risk and where to take misoprostol were causing more patients to opt for a procedural abortion. Whereas medication abortion used to represent 50 percent of all abortions at Hope Clinic, shortly after *Dobbs* the proportion dropped to 30 percent.

One of the greatest challenges Erin faces as medical director is what to do with patients who have medical complications and are not ideal candidates for an outpatient facility like Hope Clinic. In such cases the obvious medical solution would be to refer these patients for an in-hospital procedure. Even before *Dobbs*, this was often very difficult to do in conservative states, because of hospitals' reluctance to accept such patients.[8] However, Hope Clinic was fortunate because it had been able to send such patients across the river to St. Louis, which has a world-class hospital where many of Hope Clinic's doctors had privileges and longtime supportive colleagues. But after *Dobbs*, because Missouri bans abortion, it became virtually impossible for Hope Clinic to send patients with serious but not life-threatening conditions to the hospital in St. Louis.

Without the St. Louis hospital option, Erin agonized over her decision on whether to treat these patients in the clinic, saying, "I will tell you I'm a little conservative on some of these things." She explained that if performing an abortion on a medically complex patient involved a complication, it could have ramifications not only for the patient but also for Erin, compromising her ability to take care of future patients. Erin's worry was understandable because patient complications that abortion doctors face are typically scrutinized more intensively by licensing boards, the media, and others than complications other medical practitioners deal with. Anti-abortion forces are often quick to publicize or even urge lawsuits or other government action when they hear of a clinic patient being hospitalized.

When Erin suggests to patients that she would like to communicate with these patients' hometown clinicians to find out more about their medical histories, the patients often object, not wanting to reveal to anyone back home that they have traveled for abortion care. Erin was hopeful about a new program established in Illinois in 2023 that would help with some of these patients: CARLA (Complex Abortion Regional Line for Access).[9] Under this program a referral is made to an intake worker, who takes a medical history and then arranges an appointment at any one of several participating Chicago hospitals. CARLA is a prime example of the proactive steps taken in pro-choice states in the wake of *Dobbs*. For Hope Clinic patients who need hospital care, this program will undoubtedly be very beneficial, even though Chicago is several hours farther away than St. Louis.

Dealing with the small number of patients who need follow-up care after their abortion is another issue rendered more problematic for traveling patients. Erin explained, "We have patients whom we talk to on the phone that we would normally just say, 'Hey, come in. We'll see what's going on. Is your bleeding normal? Why are you having pain?'" However, in the new age of long-distance abortion travel, "They're too far away, they can't see us. So we say, 'OK, you're too far away. You need to go to the emergency room or see your gynecologist.' And they're like, 'I don't want to. I'm scared.'"

Erin additionally expressed shock at the care some of Hope Clinic's traveling patients received in their hometowns before they traveled—in many cases both serious and more simple issues have been left untreated.

For instance, with someone who has had a miscarriage, "When we say, 'This is something your gynecologist can take of,'" Erin told us, "they say, 'Oh, my gynecologist said I need to go somewhere else.' They did not need to travel six, seven, eight hours to see us for miscarriage management." Such accounts are indicative of physicians' fears in states with abortion bans of being accused of performing an abortion.

Dobbs put yet another medical issue, later abortions, on Erin's already full plate. For many years abortions after twenty weeks represented only about 1.5 percent of all abortions in the United States. With the increased difficulties of access brought by *Dobbs*, most people in abortion practice, including Erin, assumed that the increased difficulty of access would boost this percentage because of delays in getting to a clinic.

Before *Dobbs*, Hope Clinic had been caring for patients up to twenty-six weeks' gestation and would refer those over twenty-six weeks to a clinic that performed third-trimester abortions. But post-*Dobbs* Erin grew increasingly concerned about patients who were showing up after that cutoff. Erin told us, "We've been having a really hard time for our folks who are over twenty-six weeks, finding places for them to go that can see them in a fairly reasonable amount of time." The perennial shortage of clinics offering third-trimester care grew more acute when, around the time of *Dobbs*, one of the major providers of such services in New Mexico, Southwestern Women's Options, stopped offering such care.

This change spurred Erin to begin planning to raise the gestational limit at Hope Clinic to twenty-eight weeks. Erin's decision to increase Hope Clinic's offerings into a later period of gestation is consistent with a nationwide trend of clinics similarly increasing the availability of later abortions post-*Dobbs*.[10] In order to do this, Erin needed to upgrade her own skills, which she did by shadowing a colleague in another city, an innovator in third-trimester care. Staff also had to prepare and plan, as third-trimester procedures involve a longer clinic stay than medication abortion or earlier procedural abortions. The logistics of this new level of care are difficult, Erin said. "Where do they sit? What do they do? How much pain medicine do we give them? How do the nurses know when to give them the pain medicine?"

Outside of these medical concerns, another omnipresent aspect of abortion provision in surge states after *Dobbs* is the threat of increased anti-abortion targeting. Hope Clinic prepared for this possibility early. In the lead-up to the decision, the clinic met with an FBI agent, as did many other abortion providers across the country. The main purpose of the FBI visit to Hope Clinic was to train clinic personnel in the Freedom of Access to Clinic Entrances Act. The 1994 federal law, commonly known as FACE, makes it a federal crime to impede access to abortion clinics or to engage in threats or acts of violence against abortion patients or providers.[11] Erin told us that FBI agents had also been warning clinics in states where abortion would remain legal to expect a new wave of protesters when clinics closed in other states.

Hope Clinic has a particularly traumatic history with respect to anti-abortion violence. In 1982, the then owner, Hector Zevallos and his wife, Rosalie, were kidnapped by a shadowy group called the Army of God, one of the earliest instances of antiabortion terrorism in this country's history.[12] The couple were released unharmed just over a week later, but according to Erin, this incident, though it occurred forty years ago, was still part of the collective memory of the staff. Drawing on this history as well as the FBI's warnings, everyone at the clinic expected more protesters and possibly violence to come after *Dobbs*. Erin confirmed to us that, in the year of *Dobbs*, the protesters at Hope Clinic were "meaner and more aggressive" to patients and staff.

Speaking sympathetically of the staff's concerns about both security and the rise in the number of patients, Erin pointed to a shift she perceived in abortion-providing circles with respect to frontline staff. "We've spent a lot of years being patient-centered, which I think we should be." But, as a result, she acknowledged, clinics were not sufficiently staff-centered. Speculating that this shift started with the difficult working conditions during the pandemic, Erin put it in clear terms: if management is not "employee-centric at the same time we're being patient-centric, we can't take good care of the patient."

As Adrienne had done at PPRM, Hope Clinic took steps to more pro-actively address staff stress in the new *Dobbs* reality. In response to a fair amount of staff resignations, the clinic implemented increased days off, shorter working hours, resilience workshops, and improved salaries—measures that were supported by a new ownership team that took over shortly before *Dobbs*.

In this new environment of a patient surge and stress for staff, Erin was buoyed by the extraordinary amount of support patients were receiving, both financial and logistical (discussed in more detail in chapter 7). Months after *Dobbs*, Erin was still incredulous as to the outpouring of support. "The support and the amount of money that has been poured into helping these patients, at least the ones we see, get here is shocking. I'm overwhelmed. Every single patient who walks in our door from out of state that's twelve weeks or under, they're being seen at no charge, right? So, that is shocking that there's that much funding out there right now. There's organizations that are, like, 'Here is a ton of money, and it's to take care of your patients, and that patients have hotel rooms.' And these magical things are happening with flights changing, and hotel rooms, and Ubers, and car services, and private jets."

Erin explained her private jet comment further, telling us about a patient being flown to the clinic in a private plane. "She was in a domestic abuse situation and her partner had stolen her ID. She couldn't go on a domestic flight," Erin said. The support likely came from a new group formed in the wake of *Dobbs*, Elevated Access, an organization of pilots with private aircraft who volunteer to provide transportation to abortion facilities.[13]

Like almost everyone we talked to the year of *Dobbs*, Erin expressed hope that the significant amount of help available to patients, like free abortions under twelve weeks and logistical help from patient navigators, would continue. In this new world, she said, "If we're not going to be able to do it in all of the states and all of the regions [where] patients are, then funding them to get to where they can be is not the answer, but at least it's a band-aid until, hopefully, we have a better answer."

CALIFORNIA

Three days after *Dobbs*, one of Janet Jacobson's clinics received a bomb threat. The clinic was part of Planned Parenthood of Orange and San Bernardino Counties (PPOSBC) where Janet is the medical director. The call came into a clinic in San Bernardino County, one of the most conservative areas of California. Janet paraphrased the call for us: "'I put this bomb in the bathroom under the sink. It's a pipe bomb. It's going to go off, blah, blah, blah. You should all die,' that kind of thing. But then, he went into, 'I'm going to come there and just shoot all of you.' It was incredibly difficult to listen to."

Having spent her entire life fighting against gender injustice, Janet was prepared. Janet, now an obstetrician-gynecologist, fought her first gender battle in grade school when she sued to be allowed to play on the local Pop Warner football team (she won and played for three years). Later,

Janet served as a navy pilot in a combat role immediately after the combat exclusion policy for women in aviation positions was lifted. When she left the military, she entered medical school.

Her training as a pilot prepared her well. As she told the *Los Angeles Times* a few years before we spoke with her, "My time in the Navy, particularly learning to fly and being a pilot, is very similar to what it takes to survive in healthcare as a physician. You spend years training, learning, and practicing. . . . Most of the time while you are doing those things, it's pretty routine, but when something unexpected happens, all that training and practice kicks in."[14] Given this mindset, Janet had been thoughtfully preparing for *Dobbs* for several years, including preparing for antiabortion violence.

Fortunately, police responded to the bomb threat immediately, and the clinic was evacuated, including patients who were in the midst of examinations. Ironically, this particular clinic had not been offering procedural abortions at the time of the threat, though Janet planned to start doing so soon. The patients who were rushed off the exam tables and hustled outside were receiving family-planning services.

Janet and her staff were shaken by the call. Without knowing for sure, Janet suspected the caller was acting alone. "That's the person we all worry about," she said. "We have all the security in place and so on. And we have all the violent speech from protesters out there spewing hate and stuff. But those aren't the people we worry about the most. It's the one-off crazy person who is armed or has explosives."

Janet expressed admiration for the staff person at the affiliate's call center—a recent hire—who received and responded to the call. There had recently been a drill among the workers to handle bomb threats, and the new staffer did exactly as she had been instructed. "She did all the right things, kept him on the phone, went through the checklist of questions that's right by the phones." Training like this was part of the preparation for *Dobbs* that clinics had undertaken. Like other clinics in abortion-friendly locations, PPOSBC had received visits from local law enforcement and the FBI in the period leading up to the expected decision. The affiliate had been cautioned to be on alert for possible extreme activity from opponents, and PPOSBC had already beefed up security, paid for in part by a grant of several million dollars from the state of California.

An increase in antiabortion extremism has been one of the most prominent effects of *Dobbs* for Janet's clinics. When we asked Janet about the clinic protesters since *Dobbs*, she told us, "They're much more aggressive and there are many more of them." She ventured several possible reasons for this increased aggressiveness: protesters are "feeling empowered and celebrating the loss of *Roe*"; California clinics are being targeted by more extremist groups from states that no longer permit abortion services; and some of the protest is an expression of rage that abortions are still happening anywhere.

Such aggressive protests of course can be very upsetting to patients and staff alike. As Janet said with evident frustration about the impact on patients, "It kills me when a patient comes in crying, on an already difficult day." Janet herself had made the decision, because of *Dobbs*, to become more vocal than she had been in the past—including making appearances on television and writing an op-ed—a decision that caused considerable worry among her family members that doing so would put a target on Janet's back.[15] She was indeed targeted, though in a nonviolent way. One day after work she found what she sarcastically referred to as a "love note" from an abortion protester on her car in the clinic parking lot. Janet was unsettled but not at all deterred from her public-facing activities.

Janet's preparation for *Dobbs* also included making plans for a patient surge. "I know from experience," she told us, "that the switch is going to get flipped and then the flood is coming and that is not the time to start figuring things out." Janet braced for an influx of patients from Arizona, as well as patients from Texas and other parts of the country. In preparation, at one of its San Bernardino County clinics that served patients who drove across the desert from Arizona, PPOSBC engaged in extensive planning to expand its services to include procedural abortion, not just medication abortion.

Janet's ability to plan was made easier than that of medical directors of clinics elsewhere in the country because she works in a very abortion-friendly state. Janet had participated in the California Future of Abortion Council, a group convened by California Governor Gavin Newsom in anticipation of *Dobbs* overruling *Roe*. The group's efforts were successful; the state legislature passed many of its suggested measures to support both patients and abortion providers.[16]

Another positive factor for Janet was that some of PPOSBC's nine facilities (with one more in the planning stage when we first spoke with her) are located in areas of considerable wealth in Orange County, which makes for a very generous donor base. Janet proudly told us that even before *Dobbs*,

PPOSBC never turned away a patient if they could not afford an abortion. She then elaborated on the various supports put into place in anticipation of *Dobbs*, much of which was possible only because of the organization's resources: "We now have seven-days-a-week coverage with the patient navigator. We have contracts with various hotels near our surgical sites. We have arrangements now with ride shares. We have corporate accounts with airlines." Remarking that the great majority of her patients drove to the clinic and that actually very few patients made use of flight vouchers, she also mentioned a new program that supplied gas cards.

With a large staff across many sites, Janet had the flexibility to switch people around to meet shifting needs in light of the changing landscape. Janet said of her staff, with respect to anticipating what the *Dobbs* decision might mean, "I think they're excited to be part of the solution, just like they were excited to be open during the pandemic when all the other doctors' offices were closed, and nobody could get care. I think they are excited to do that, and then it is my job to make it sustainable for them."

Janet's approach to making things sustainable for her staff was to periodically rotate them out of a hectic schedule that operated seven days a week, starting at 6:30 a.m., even before the increase in patients that was anticipated to come after *Dobbs*. Though she told us of efforts to avoid burnout of her clinicians by limiting the amount of abortion care they performed, she took pains to schedule a few hours a week of abortion provision for herself, as a relief from administrative work. "I have to keep that connection, so I can keep my sanity."

Still another advantage PPOSBC had in planning for *Dobbs* was that its California location meant there was an abundant supply of doctors and other clinicians trained in abortion care. Six major academic medical centers in the state not only offer abortion training but also host the Complex Family Planning Fellowship, which trains in methods of later abortions.[17] The "luxury," as Janet put it, of having seven fellowship-trained physicians on her staff is particularly important because even though these procedures are rare, several of PPOSBC's clinics perform abortion through twenty-three weeks and six days of gestation. Abortions in the second trimester of pregnancy are typically performed over two days. But even before *Dobbs* the provider community had begun to expect greatly increased patient travel, particularly by those seeking second-trimester care. Consequently, some physicians, particularly those within fellowship circles, developed methods of performing these abortions in one day. Janet believed that this level of advanced training of her staff would be consequential, as many of those needing such services post-*Dobbs* were predicted to be travelers for whom an extra day away from home would be costly in terms of lodging, lost wages, childcare, and other expenses.

PPOSBC also had an advantage in the provision of earlier abortions. For first-trimester abortions, California law allows advanced practice clinicians—physician assistants, nurse midwives, and nurse practitioners—to offer both medication abortion and first-trimester procedural abortions. Janet told us that a number of providers in states that now have bans have contacted her about the possibility of working at her affiliate—but, she said, "I have no place to put them!" The staffing challenge for many providers was to find support staff such as medical assistants, not doctors or advanced practice clinicians.

When *Dobbs* hit, PPOSBC saw an increase in out-of-state patients, but not as large as expected. Janet had planned for 160 out-of-state patients per month, but six months after *Dobbs*, PPOSBC was averaging about 45. Arizona clinics did shut down soon after *Dobbs* but then reopened shortly thereafter as a result of a favorable state court ruling.[18] Also, most abortion patients in states with bans, disproportionately in the South and Midwest, preferred to drive to places more conveniently located than California, such as Colorado, Illinois, and New Mexico, and that eased the pressure on PPOSBC.

The Guttmacher Institute's study of post-*Dobbs* abortion travel confirmed what Janet experienced. California saw only a small increase of abortions after *Dobbs*, and only 16 percent of those were from travelers, compared to New Mexico's whopping 220 percent increase, of which 87 percent were from travelers.[19] Nonetheless, even though the increase wasn't as much as expected, Janet and her staff continue to be proud to serve these new patients who are fleeing abortion bans elsewhere.

WASHINGTON STATE

When we first spoke to Mercedes Sanchez in early 2022, she was predicting a "tsunami" of out-of-state patients coming to her clinics. Mercedes was the director of development, communications, and community education and outreach at Cedar River Clinics, a network of three independent abortion clinics in Washington State. As a second-trimester abortion provider, Cedar River Clinics already saw a considerable number of patients from states across the country that had restrictive laws around gestational limits. Her clinics even see a steady stream of patients from Alaska because they accept Alaska Medicaid and clinics in that state are hard to access. Commenting on Alaska patients flying to Washington for abortions, Mercedes made us laugh when she quipped, "Sarah Palin may be able to see Russia from her front porch, but most people in Alaska can't see a clinic from theirs."

Mercedes took one of the more unusual routes to abortion work. She attributes the beginnings of her path toward a career in this field to her experience, as a Catholic child, of preparing for her first communion. "We did classes before our first communion ceremony. And I remember one class, they brought in what I would later learn was a group of [people who were antiabortion]. And they wanted us to write prayers or poems about all the dead babies from abortions. Even as a little kid, and not really knowing what it is," Mercedes said she thought, "'This sounds wrong to me.' Kids, I think, have BS meters. And clearly, this is stuck in my memory for decades. And I remember not doing it."

Years later, as a young adult volunteering for a variety of liberal causes, she went with a friend to a local abortion clinic in Santa Fe, New Mexico, to serve as a clinic escort and was dismayed to see protesters screaming at patients. This experience led to a flashback: "I remember thinking back to my first communion and thinking that the visitors "must've been the people over there." This realization, coupled with eventual volunteer work at a Seattle clinic, led to a decision to work in the field of abortion provision. She joined Cedar River Clinics in 2012, where she has taken on ever-increasing responsibility.[20]

Working in Washington for her entire career in the field of abortion, Mercedes has had the luxury of being in a very pro-choice state. Recently, that has meant strong support from the governor and the Democrat-led state legislature. Governor Jay Inslee signed a measure keeping abortion facilities open during the height of the Covid-19 pandemic, declaring them to be "essential healthcare" at a time when governors in conservative states were using the pandemic as an excuse to shut clinics down.[21] He also took the lead in organizing several other abortion-supportive states to mount a federal court challenge to the FDA's overregulation of mifepristone, a lawsuit for which Mercedes and her colleagues were consulted by the governor's staff as the challenge was being prepared. After *Dobbs*, Mercedes told us, several elected officials, including the governor, reached out and came to tour Cedar River's main clinic in Renton, a suburb of Seattle.

One of the major adjustments that Cedar River made in anticipation of an expected post-*Dobbs* increased patient load was to expand options at its Yakima clinic to include procedural abortion. Yakima is two hours east of Seattle and three hours from the Idaho border. Previously, the clinic had only done telehealth medication abortion, so expanding care at that facility made procedural abortion more accessible to people in the eastern part of the state. Mercedes told us that Cedar River first rented space in Yakima in 1979. Once there, she said, "our clinic was the focus of blockades in the 1980s, and we did lawsuits against antiabortion groups, and the settlement money (as well as donations) helped us to buy our building there." The clinic had stopped providing services there in 2010, but the building then was repurposed as Cedar River's business center. Mercedes was very proud of how the Yakima facility had come full circle back to providing all levels of abortion care.

Dobbs, though completely expected, was nonetheless deeply upsetting for Mercedes and her staff. "It was heartbreak—and then it was just resolve, like we just have to get back to work. We were providing services that day, so the focus was the patients." In the immediate aftermath of the decision, besides being buoyed by the abovementioned visits from the governor and other elected officials, Mercedes was also gratified by the numerous gestures of support from the local community: many people offered to volunteer; a brewery gave the clinic naming rights to a new craft beer; a bakery designated profits from a favored item for the clinic; and flowers and food were sent to the clinic by various businesses and individuals. As Mercedes said, "When we're exhausted, it's really nice to see that individuals in our community are supporting us."

Six months after *Dobbs*, Mercedes acknowledged that the "tsunami" that she had earlier predicted would emerge if *Roe* fell had thus far failed to materialize, saying, "My newest sound bite is, when an abortion ban goes into effect, not everyone is pregnant at the same time. I say it's more like the rising tide. I think we're just going to keep seeing more patients unless something happens. So, more like a rising flood situation than huge waves and surges." And Mercedes was right. Although Washington didn't see the massive increase of out-of-state patients that Colorado and New Mexico did, it did see more than 1,400 people traveling from out of state in 2022, a 46 percent increase from 2021.[22] Out of an abundance of legal caution, Cedar River is not publicly discussing the increase in the number of patients or which states they are coming from. But Mercedes told us, "It is a truly significant increase for us, and it is patients from around the country, not just neighboring states. As bans and restrictions went into effect, the flood waters rose higher."

Mercedes raised two concerns regarding the increased number of patients going forward: sufficient staff and sufficient funds to meet the increased patient load. The staffing challenges, mentioned by virtually every clinic director we spoke to, involved hiring medical assistants, nurses, and mid-level administrators. Medical assistants, as Mercedes put it, "are like gold." She wistfully mentioned to us how a local medical clinic affiliated with a major medical center in Seattle offered a $5,000 signing bonus to medical assistants, money Cedar River could not match. Mercedes also mentioned contacting twenty-six colleagues in the area for help in locating a development and marketing associate and receiving no referrals.

These hard-to-fill positions posed an interesting contrast to the difficulties clinics faced in earlier years: finding clinicians to perform abortions. Though this problem has not entirely disappeared, in some liberal areas there actually is an oversupply of providers, and Seattle is one of them. Mercedes quoted a colleague who likes to say, "You can't swing a cat without hitting an abortion provider in Seattle."

Funding is another real challenge, causing Mercedes to quip, "Our safety net has holes in it." She worried that there would simply not be enough money to accommodate the additional staff that needed to be hired, nor to offer reduced or free abortions to patients who cannot afford them. Her concerns were partially met by a shared grant of $7.4 million that the state provided to abortion clinics as a belated payment from state Covid funding. Money concerns also abated somewhat after generous donations for patients from the area's abortion fund, the Northwest Abortion Access Fund. The fund was especially helpful in paying for travel costs and assistance with abortion costs for those who traveled to Cedar River Clinics. Still, adequate funding is a constant worry for Mercedes and almost every other abortion provider we spoke to.

STAFFING THE ABORTION WORKFORCE

Dobbs has made staffing a major concern of almost everyone working at abortion clinics. To be sure, the concerns are different depending on where the clinic is located. Those in states where abortion is now banned worried about the employment prospects of staff who had worked in their clinics, some for several decades. Those working in states where surges were expected, like the people in this chapter, were frantically trying to hire enough new employees to meet the expected flood of new patients coming from states with abortion bans.

Solving the staffing problem is Mary Frank's main job in her work with the National Abortion Federation (NAF), and she is one of the savviest people in the country about abortion staffing. Mary has deep experience in abortion work, having administered several clinics and long served as a consultant in this field. In her current position she leads NAF's Clinic Abortion Staffing Solutions project (CASS), which helps match clinics needing staff and people seeking work in the field of abortion provision.

Mary experienced her own deluge after *Dobbs*, though a different type than providers faced. On the day *Dobbs* was decided CASS received more than triple the number of inquiry emails it usually receives per day—sixty-five instead of the usual twenty. The emails were from people "asking could they help, they want to help, how can they help?" This barrage of inquiries persisted for several days afterward.

Part of Mary's responsibilities at NAF also include running the Training Institute, a network of several regional facilities that offer training in abortion care. Some of the emails Mary received on that day were also from physicians and advance practice clinicians asking for abortion training.

As Mary saw it, the two greatest post-*Dobbs* staffing needs in surge states were going to be for doctors trained to perform abortions past twenty weeks in gestation and registered nurses and other frontline staff such as medical assistants and receptionists. In fact, even before *Dobbs*, the pandemic had made clear to her how desperate clinics were to hire the latter, and she had built up a database of about two hundred such individuals, hoping to place them.

Each group posed its own challenges. With hiring doctors to work in a new state that was seeing an increase in patients, the main stumbling block is obtaining licensing in the new state. Once they obtain their license, they face the complicated issue of whether performing abortions in a state where it is legal will affect medical licenses they continue to hold from states that now ban abortion. Some abortion-friendly states have moved to protect providers in this situation, but as a general matter this issue remains unresolved.[23]

Another challenge for Mary with this first group of staff was that most of the doctors who contacted CASS immediately after *Dobbs* did not want to completely relocate, but rather preferred to travel to provide care. But to make it worth it for the clinic to hire the doctor, providers must be able to travel a significant amount. As Mary said, "Unfortunately, offering to help just a small number of times per year is not that helpful."

With respect to the challenges posed by nonlicensed staff, Mary conveyed the pain that many clinic directors in states with bans now in place felt about laying off frontline employees. She told us of efforts to work with this group, for example by pointing to retraining opportunities through various government-sponsored workplace development programs. However, it is easy to imagine that someone in a very conservative state whose résumé shows that the only previous job experience was working in an abortion clinic for years could have trouble being hired elsewhere in that state.

Mary explained that another challenge for frontline staff was that even if they were willing to relocate, clinics were usually not in a position to pay the expenses for them to do so or to travel, whereas generally they were willing to pay travel or relocation costs for doctors, since abortion-providing clinicians brought in the most revenue.

When we checked in with Mary in 2023, we found that what she had anticipated with respect to workforce issues had come to pass. "Demand is down for physicians who only provide to fourteen weeks" she told us. As she predicted, the greatest need was for those who were trained to perform abortions later in pregnancy. Echoing Mercedes's lament about hiring challenges in Washington State, Mary said, "Abortion clinics are competing for staff with general healthcare organizations [and] our clinics struggle to compete with wages for these workers."

SERVING EVERYONE WHO SHOWS UP

Despite all of the challenges the providers in this chapter and others like them throughout the country have faced post-*Dobbs*, they have done everything in their power to continue to care not only for the patients they have always served but also for new patients traveling from far away. These providers know they are a key part of the post-*Dobbs* abortion ecosystem and an important reason abortions continue to be available despite the Supreme Court's ruling.

Perhaps speaking for all the providers facing this surge, Janet told us that on the day *Dobbs* was decided, she and her staff felt "this amazing grief . . . followed very shortly by anger." But their grief and rage were accompanied by another emotion: resolve. "And that's what I've been telling the staff," Janet said. "'You know what? We're just going to do what we can and see who we can see. We're going to get whoever we can here. We're not turning anyone away.'"

CHAPTER SIX

PILLS

We have the tools to create a meaningful landscape of abortion access in post-Dobbs America, but we need to dramatically increase the level of participation. We need people to stop seeing abortion as something that they can only have if a court gives them the right to it and start seeing access as something which fundamentally belongs to all of us.

—AMELIA BONOW, Shout Your Abortion

The antiabortion movement and the abortion rights and justice movement don't agree on much, but after *Dobbs*, one point of agreement was the new importance of abortion pills. Simply put, in 2023, 63 percent of abortions in the United States were in the form of medication abortion (up from 53 percent in 2020), showing the clear importance of abortion pills to abortion seekers and providers.[1]

Because of the importance of medication abortion, much of the antiabortion movement is laser-focused on pills. Students for Life called abortion pills "the new frontier of abortion," the National Right to Life Committee said that pills meant the movement needed "a new approach," and Americans United for Life said that they are the "No. 1 issue for those who desire to protect life."[2] They saw the writing on the wall in a post-*Roe* country. People will find ways to obtain abortion pills to terminate pregnancies in places where abortion became illegal . . . and it would be hard, if not impossible, to stop.

Focusing attention on abortion pills is not exactly new. Long before abortion pills were first presented to the Food and Drug Administration for approval in 1996, the antiabortion movement had been working to stop what it considered "chemical warfare on the unborn."[3] Its efforts succeeded in delaying the introduction of abortion pills into the American market but were not successful in ultimately blocking them. In 2000, over a decade and a half after initial testing in other countries, eight to twelve years after other countries approved it, and almost four years after the initial approval request, the FDA approved mifepristone for use to terminate a pregnancy.

For over two decades, Americans have had abortion pills available to them. As discussed in the introduction, the regimen approved by the FDA involves two pills, mifepristone and misoprostol. The FDA approved mifepristone for abortion in 2000; misoprostol is approved for ulcer treatment and is used off-label for various obstetric purposes, including abortion. The two drugs are taken in succession, with different providers varying both the time between pills and the total dosages. In most pregnancies, mifepristone ends the growth of the fetus, and misoprostol induces uterine contractions to expel the pregnancy tissue. The entire process can last anywhere from twenty-four to seventy-two hours, but light bleeding can continue for up to a few weeks. The FDA has approved the use of abortion pills through eleven weeks of pregnancy, but they can be safely and effectively used even later into pregnancy.[4]

Abortion pills have become increasingly popular as a method of abortion. Because the process is completed outside a medical facility, women using them are able to end their pregnancy in the privacy and comfort of their own chosen surroundings and with people of their own choosing (if any) accompanying them.

The number of people using abortion pills has increased in part because of one of the most significant changes in abortion pills since their approval in 2000. Until 2020, the FDA required people to obtain abortion pills in person from a certified provider. When the pandemic hit, women continued to get pregnant and want abortions, but they sought to do so with the least amount of contact with others as possible so as to lower their risk of being infected with Covid-19. Other areas of medicine faced the same issue and as a result saw a rise in telehealth. The FDA facilitated that increase by relaxing in-person distribution rules during the pandemic; however, that change did not cover abortion pills. A federal lawsuit to force the FDA to relax the requirement for obtaining mifepristone in person was initially successful in July 2020, but the Supreme Court reinstated the in-person requirement in January 2021.[5]

But when Joe Biden succeeded Donald Trump as president, the FDA, reflecting the transition from an antiabortion administration to a pro-choice one, changed its approach in April 2021, announcing that it was temporarily lifting the in-person requirement due to the pandemic; in December it announced it was doing so permanently. These changes paved the way for people to obtain abortion pills by mail directly from a certified provider or, with a prescription, from a certified mail-order pharmacy. In January 2023, the FDA released new rules outlining how mail-order and brick-and-mortar pharmacies could get certified to dispense mifepristone to people with a prescription.[6]

Most of these rule changes occurred just before we started conducting the interviews for this book. There is no doubt that the increased ease of access for lawfully obtaining abortion pills has contributed to alleviating much of the predicted disaster from the Supreme Court's overturning *Roe*. Moreover, beyond the FDA-approved market for abortion pills, informal networks, international pharmacies, and online stores offering abortion pills for no- or low-cost have proliferated. Because of these changes as well as the general trajectory of greater use of pills by patients, almost everyone we talked with for this book mentioned pills in some way when they discussed how abortion care was changing because of the overturning of *Roe*.

In particular, the five people featured in this chapter talked almost exclusively about the role of abortion pills in a post-*Roe* future. Together, they paint a picture of the various strategies being employed to deliver more pills to more patients, including for those who now live in states where abortion is banned. They take different approaches—some within the already-existing medical establishment, some pushing the boundaries of that establishment, and some almost completely ignoring them—but they share the same view: abortion pills, although not a complete solution to the problems created by overturning *Roe*, are a critical part of making sure people can get the care they need in a country where abortion bans are proliferating.

EXPANDING TELEHEALTH

Traditional abortion clinics that offer various types of abortion methods have long offered abortion pills as an option for their patients. As more and more patients wanted abortion pills rather than procedural abortion, pills-only clinics began to appear. For these clinics and other primary-care healthcare providers who could offer abortion pills as part of their practices, ending a pregnancy with pills rather than a procedure became the dominant form of abortion in this country.

Once abortion pills could be delivered to patients by mail, providers were given even more room for innovation. Jamie Phifer—a family doctor who is the founder and medical director of Abortion On Demand, AOD for short—tried to make abortion pills available in as many states as lawfully possible. Once the FDA relaxed the in-person requirement for mifepristone in 2021, Jamie created AOD to bring telehealth abortion to more people in more states.

Her model is straightforward. A patient fills out an online intake questionnaire that is reviewed to make sure that the patient meets AOD's basic requirements—a positive pregnancy test, eighteen years of age or older, under fifty-six days since last menstrual period, and a mailing address in a state where telehealth abortion is legal and AOD operates. There are also screening questions to weed out people who are at risk of ectopic pregnancy or who have other medically disqualifying conditions.

If, based on answers on the questionnaire, the patient qualifies for a medication abortion, AOD arranges a video session between the patient and the provider. Patients can be anywhere in the US when they fill out the online intake form, but for the video call the patient must be physically located in a state where telehealth abortion is legal and AOD operates. To further protect itself and the patient, AOD does not allow patients to use post office boxes or mail forwarding. Jamie recognized that this is a conservative approach, especially in the face of the loss of access post-*Dobbs*, but told us that she made this decision in order to avoid risk to everyone involved. "The whole model is designed so that I can say, on my end, that the abortion is occurring in one of the states in which telemedicine abortion is fully legal. I need to do everything on my end to show that."

The video call is a one-on-one consult with a licensed clinician. The calls tend to last between eight and twelve minutes, with the clinician answering any questions the patient has. Most patient concerns are addressed in a pre-recorded counseling video they have already watched that covers the basics, so the provider calls are relatively quick. "Most of our patients don't require a lot of clinician time," Jamie said. "I think that people don't need their hands held, and I don't think they need to be babysat over it." Once the patient's consult is complete and she has consented to the abortion, AOD works with three different pharmacies who ship pills to the patient's mailing address for the patient to take once they are received.

When Jamie started AOD, she had hopes of bringing the model to as many states as possible. When we first talked with her in early 2022, she was operating in twenty-one states and hoped to expand into more. She had the experience and background to do so. Prior to starting AOD, Jamie had been working for a national telehealth company that was not involved with abortion care. As part of this work, she obtained licenses to practice medicine in all fifty states so she could care for patients everywhere.

But abortion care was her passion. In medical school in Florida, Jamie was introduced to the organization Medical Students for Choice by a friend who attended school in North Carolina. Her friend invited Jamie to North Carolina for a chapter meeting, and Jamie drove the nine hours to attend. The meeting made an impression on her: when she returned to Florida, she started a chapter at her own school. Soon after, in 2009, George Tiller, the high-profile Kansas doctor who provided abortion care throughout pregnancy, was assassinated by an antiabortion extremist. To Jamie, and so many other abortion providers, his work and that of others like him was inspiring.

Jamie also realized that she had a special affinity for this work. "I do not like continuity of care," she said, using the medical term for long-term, ongoing management of health issues by clinicians. "I think my skill set is that I'm very good at making people feel like they're the only person in the world for ten minutes. Just ten minutes. And that's a great skill to have as an abortion provider."

After medical school Jamie completed her residency in Seattle where she was grateful to have many opportunities to train in abortion care, including second- and third-trimester care, which she described as her passion. Once she finished her residency, she began traveling to Florida and Montana to provide abortion care. When the pandemic hit she couldn't travel any longer, so she started her work with the national telehealth company that gave her the skills to start AOD and combine her passion for abortion care with her new telehealth experience.

Developing innovative care models seems to be baked into Jamie's being. She explained that ideally she "would love for abortion care to be incorporated into primary care." But she believes we are decades away from that model being adopted on a mass scale because of how siloed abortion is in medicine. But, she told us, she actually likes "that abortion care has been outside of the medical industrial complex for all these years. It's been an opportunity for me to be creative as a physician, from an operational standpoint, to reflect on just how someone's experience is from the beginning to end. That's what I love about AOD. I just wanted to build things and see if they would work."

This quality put Jamie in a great position to be both prepared for and nimble in the face of the Supreme Court's overturning of *Roe*. For instance, after *Dobbs* was decided, Jamie wound down her operations for Georgia patients because she anticipated that legal restrictions would soon be in effect there.

At the same time, she began to implement a unique plan she had for Pennsylvania and Washington, DC, that put a creative twist on the AOD model that reflected the particular needs in those places. Initially, Jamie told us, even though abortion is legal, both Pennsylvania's and DC's abortion laws made it difficult for a virtual clinic to operate. So instead of using the usual AOD model to serve patients in those places, Jamie innovated. Under this new model, AOD providers conducted the video counseling call while the patient was in Pennsylvania or DC but had the pharmacy send the pills to a location (such as a mailing center that receives packages for people) over the border into a state where AOD can provide abortions—New Jersey or Maryland for Pennsylvania and Maryland for DC.

Jamie adapted this post-*Dobbs* model based on what "happens all the time" with telemedicine for people who live on the border of two states. "Like patients who might work in Philadelphia and live in New Jersey. If they're having their blood pressure medications managed and they're doing their video visit on their lunch break in Philadelphia, presumably their physician is licensed in Pennsylvania, but they might have their blood pressure medication sent to them in New Jersey." Even though this new service delivery model didn't make up for the post-*Dobbs* loss of patients in the one state where she had to stop providing care, Georgia, it did help patients in other states.

Consistent with Jamie's overall philosophy, AOD is pushing boundaries with this new model but also taking a conservative approach. For instance, Pennsylvania is the only state for which AOD requires patients to have a state ID. Jamie recognized that this means people from, say, Ohio (a state with an abortion ban when we talked with Jamie in 2022), couldn't drive across the border into Pennsylvania to use AOD's services. Though many people in the movement are promoting pills for traveling patients, Jamie was concerned that a patient returning to a hostile state such as Ohio in the middle of the regimen would face too much risk: A small percentage of abortion-pill users experience continued pregnancies or incomplete abortions requiring further care; if that occurs back home in a state with an abortion ban, Jamie was concerned, there might be legal problems for the patient or AOD.

Despite these limitations, Jamie thinks her model still benefits post-*Dobbs* travelers. Providing care for early-first-trimester Pennsylvanians needing abortions can free up appointments in the state's brick-and-mortar clinics to care for out-of-state travelers seeking in-person care in Pennsylvania.

For other states that Jamie perceived as less risky, AOD does care for travelers. Jamie tells patients, "If you are traveling for care, we would highly encourage you to seek in-person services for a procedure or to stay in that state until your pregnancy symptoms are clearly gone." If a patient needs follow-up care in a state AOD serves, AOD can help coordinate that care. But if the patient travels back to a state where abortion is banned and has a medical issue after the abortion is complete, Jamie said, "we can ask that they seek emergency services, but we cannot coordinate their care in a restricted state."

When we talked with Jamie at the end of 2022, she was about to implement a new model for Kansas. Jamie explained that even though abortion is legal in Kansas, the situation there is legally complicated for a variety of reasons, so AOD has to take extra precautions. She didn't want to go into details with us, but she said that because Kansas is surrounded by states with bans, "we take a very conservative approach to where the abortion occurs."

Now that abortion is illegal in Texas, providing care for people physically located in Kansas is important for patients coming from eastern Texas, as Kansas is the closest state where abortion remains legal. "I think we're going to get a lot of people who are willing to drive to Kansas and stay two or three days for a telehealth abortion. And so, we're going to have to do a lot more phone calls, back and forth, with patients to make sure that we're following the law in Kansas if they're traveling."

Jamie noted several other challenges since *Dobbs*. One is that more patients are trying to mask their location, such as by purchasing post office boxes. AOD will not serve these patients. Jamie estimated that about half of the patients contacting AOD immediately after *Dobbs* "were very clearly not in one of the states that we could serve." Dealing with those patients took a lot of staffing time, but she and her colleagues would try to provide them with resources that might help them find care while explaining that AOD is not an option for them.

Jamie worries about quality of care in this new post-*Dobbs* market. She is concerned that well-meaning providers are going to begin offering medication abortion drugs online without truly understanding the legal risk and logistical complexity of delivering this model of care. She is especially concerned about people who previously were not abortion providers but had experience with telemedicine who don't realize how different abortion practice is, particularly the regulations and the public scrutiny. "I think that there's folks who think they're doing well, who are going to screw it up and get themselves in trouble, which then gets us in trouble."

An even greater worry is that opportunists will enter the market: "There's going to be bad actors trying to make a buck, and there'll be a lot of those." Immediately after *Dobbs* was decided, the telehealth abortion landscape became populated with many venture capitalists trying to profit from this new legal environment.[7] Many of these were reputable doctors trying to find their way into the market, but others were not—for instance, websites popped up selling fake abortion pills. Jamie speculated this may well be the antiabortion movement "selling fake pills as a means of stirring up doubt about legitimate telemedicine providers."

Jamie positions AOD completely differently: a provider of high-quality care with a conservative legal approach so that people can point to her service as the "standard of care" in the field. At the same time, Jamie recognizes the upside to having so many other telehealth abortion providers post-*Dobbs*—it helps to normalize her model. "I think it's good for the patient because there are so many players," she said. "We're not just one of two providers in a couple states and the patients are trying to decide whether we're sketchy or whether telehealth abortion is really a thing."

As Jamie and AOD continue to navigate the post-*Dobbs* landscape, she knows there are still areas for improvement, saying "'Rising tides lifts all boats' only helps if you have a fucking boat." What she means is that the promise of telemedicine abortion, with all the money and tech being poured into it, won't be realized until there is more support for what the patients need. Right now, there are still language, technology, financial, and legal barriers for too many people who want abortion care, so even if innovation and funding pour into the telehealth space, not everyone will be helped.

As Jamie looks into the future, she hopes to expand her care model to incorporate more languages and a greater number of partnerships to reach people who need care. She knows that to do so will require her to adapt to the constantly changing landscape. For instance, in 2023, after we finished our last interview with Jamie and after there were new legal developments in those states, AOD was able to change its service models for Pennsylvania and Kansas to allow for easier patient access.

MOBILE ABORTION CLINICS

Meg Sasse Stern is part of a different effort to expand the reach of abortion pills by pushing the boundaries of traditional clinic models. In mid-2022 she became the community engagement and partnerships manager of Just The Pill. That organization started in 2021 as a telehealth option for abortion pills but has evolved to include trying a new approach that has particular importance post-*Dobbs*: mobile vans to deliver pills to people in remote locations, especially those near states with abortion bans. Meg was hired in mid-2022 to help make this vision a reality.

Meg, who fittingly showed us, during one of our interviews, a tattoo of two abortion pills on her arm, is a veteran of the abortion world, someone who has creatively used a variety of skills to ensure access for the most marginalized people. As a teenager growing up in Louisville, Kentucky, she was part of an antiauthoritarian, anticapitalist, antipatriarchy crowd. She and her friends—"the punks, the goths, the queers, that's me"—began escorting at the local abortion clinic in 1999. Meg loved it. She could be her "smelly and angry and sleep-deprived" teenage self on the sidewalk putting her body between the aggressive protesters and the patients—"be the sand in the gears" of the antiabortion movement. Meg and her colleagues were on the sidewalk as escorts until the Louisville clinic shut down right after *Dobbs*.

In 2011, Meg joined the board of a local organization, the Kentucky Health Justice Network. Along with training and supporting clinic escorts, the group assisted abortion patients financially and helped coordinate and provide their transportation. She became an employee and remained one until the year we interviewed her, 2022. Meg also did contract work for the National Network of Abortion Funds (NNAF) and Ibis Reproductive Health, a reproductive health research organization. In fact, when we first talked with Meg in early 2022, she was working with NNAF on a project to create a comprehensive regional abortion practical support and funding network, work that did not progress beyond the pilot phase, despite the importance for coordinated patient access post-*Dobbs*.

When she started with Just The Pill in mid-2022, Meg brought to the organization's work her long history with the movement, her various skill sets, and her radical approach to abortion access and justice. Her role was to operationalize the organization's new plan to add mobile abortion clinics to its already thriving virtual-care options. The virtual-care model Just The Pill had been using doesn't differ much from the AOD model described earlier: patients connect with Just The Pill virtually and have a remote telehealth appointment with a clinician. Then Just The Pill mails pills to patients in one of the four states it serves—Colorado, Minnesota, Montana, and Wyoming.

The mobile abortion clinic model expands Just The Pill's reach to those who can't have pills mailed to them for one reason or another. For instance, a patient who lives in a state with an abortion ban couldn't receive pills without the provider and the patient possibly running afoul of the law. Or, even if a patient lives in a state where abortion remains legal, she might feel that pills delivered by mail would arrive too late or not be private given other members of her household. Just The Pill's mobile clinic is designed to help with these problems and any others that make complete virtual care difficult. To address these hurdles, Just The Pill has developed a few different unmarked mobile vehicles that bring abortion pills to people in private locations.

Just The Pill offers an innovative model of care modeled on community-based "accompaniment" often encountered in the Global South.[8] Sometimes referred to as "wraparound support," this care model helps meet people's needs beyond the financial cost of care and actively supports the person with transportation, lodging, meals, childcare, and more. Patients travel to a location where the van is located and have an appointment with a clinician at a nearby building—a community center, a church, sometimes nearby office space—where there's a waiting area with a restroom, food, coffee, and maybe crafts to pass the time. When it's their time to see the provider, the patients go to a private room for their virtual or in-person consultation, depending on the arrangements for that particular clinic session. Once that is complete, the patient can pick up the medicine at the van, which is waiting outside.

Meg's role with the mobile clinics is mostly operational and logistical. Part of that is working with the communities where the van might go. She knows that not all communities would want an abortion van rolling into their town and seeing patients, saying, "We know that we can't just go into communities without an invitation." Just The Pill has to be intentional about going where they are wanted or invited. Part of Meg's job now is to work with groups within the various towns Just The Pill is considering sending its van and other services, to try to ease their entry into the community.

The ultimate goal with the mobile clinic is to make abortions as accessible as possible for people who want them, especially now that abortion is illegal in broad swaths of the country. Meg said that Just The Pill wants to "go where it's easy for people to get to us. We definitely want to get closer to borders of states with severe restrictions."

With that goal in mind, Meg and Just The Pill have many ideas for the mobile clinic that are outside the traditional medical delivery model. For instance, Meg suggested bringing the van to a hotel parking lot after arranging for traveling patients to get rooms at that particular hotel. The patients can have their virtual appointments while in the hotel room and then walk into the parking lot where the van will be waiting for them with pills. Or parking the van at an airport, for those who need to travel by air to get to a more hospitable location. Or even creating a mobile clinic in which procedural abortions can be performed. Just The Pill has already outfitted a van as a clinic for procedures, but when we last talked with her at the end of 2022, Meg said the organization had not yet started offering this service. For all of these service models, Meg would love to raise enough money—another part of her job—"to guarantee no-cost abortions for people who are coming from places where it has been outlawed."

Mobile clinics still have to comply with all of the legal requirements of the state and locality where they operate. But Meg's and the organization's attitude is that within this legal framework there are plenty of opportunities to push the boundaries and take risks. At the end of 2022, Meg told us, "I'm so frustrated right now. My big gripe about this moment is how, and maybe it's just what I'm hearing because of the spaces I'm in, how there's still this huge fear about liability from people who can take some fucking risks but are too caught up in being worried about worst-case scenarios and what might happen." As Meg sees it, this fear of risk-taking is the opposite of what should be happening right now: providers should be willing to do whatever they can to make space for people to get care. Because this is the approach Just The Pill is taking in the post-*Dobbs* era, Meg is excited to be a part of this effort.

Six months after *Dobbs*, the mobile clinic was traveling only within Colorado but had been in Minnesota at times during the year. The hope was to expand its reach to other states, possibly Illinois and New Mexico. Just The Pill's original service model—virtual care and mailing of abortion pills—also continued to operate in Minnesota, Montana, and Wyoming. Over the course of 2022, for all different models of care, Just The Pill provided three thousand abortions, which Meg was proud of given that it was a new model of care and that many of the patients served were from states where abortion was now banned.

NEW MODELS BEYOND THE CLINIC

These care models are extensions of the traditional healthcare system in the United States, in which a licensed provider works within legal boundaries to deliver care to patients who are allowed to access that care. It should come as no surprise that after *Dobbs*, many people are pushing the envelope beyond this model. Because of the creativity of people in the movement and the ease with which pills and drugs of all types have consistently avoided detection and elimination (just think of the lack of success of the War on Drugs), there is a growing sense that, even if antiabortion efforts were able somehow to stop legal distribution, abortion pills can't be stopped.[9]

Perhaps the biggest threat to abortion bans is for people in states where abortion is legal to mail abortion pills to people who live in states with bans. Linda Prine spent 2022 trying to figure out how to do just that. Linda is a family medicine doctor practicing in New York State who was on the verge of retiring when *Dobbs* changed her mind. As an abortion provider, she has worn many hats: she works with the international organization Aid Access; until the end of 2022 she provided care for a clinic in New Mexico; she works closely with the website Plan C (discussed later in this chapter) on issues relating to telehealth abortion standards and practice; and she works with the Miscarriage and Abortion Hotline (the Hotline, for short).

Her work with the Hotline was what propelled her into her late-career post-*Dobbs* activism. In 2019, she helped start the Hotline with another doctor. The Hotline is a resource for people who have questions about managing abortions or miscarriages. It has a website with information for people who are using abortion pills but also has an eighteen-hour-a-day phone number where medical professionals are available to answer people's questions via either phone calls or texts.

Linda told us that when she and her colleague started the Hotline, "The lawyers we met with pretty universally told us that it was a bad idea and that we could get in some kind of trouble," but they forged ahead anyway. The Hotline collects no personal information from callers and only asks for information that is needed to give necessary medical advice. Most callers' questions are about levels of bleeding or cramping associated with using abortion pills. Linda explained, "Medication abortion is so safe that it's extremely rare for us to even have to send somebody to the hospital. Ninety-nine percent of the time we are reassuring people that everything is going fine medically. In the rare times we do need to advise someone to seek in-person care, our advice centers around how to discuss what is happening as a miscarriage [not as an abortion]. In other words, it's the legal risks, not the medical risks, that people using pills by mail may encounter."

When the Hotline first started, callers mostly asked where they could find pills. Linda and her colleagues would refer those callers to Plan C, a website that offers extensive information on this topic. As people found and began using pills in greater numbers, the Hotline workers realized that some people taking pills want contact with a healthcare provider to help them through the process. Post-*Dobbs*, the problem for people who were using pills without a provider's supervision is that there was often no one left locally in states with abortion bans to turn to as everyone feared criminal charges. The Hotline filled that gap in care and now fields calls and texts from increasing numbers of people every month.

Hearing of the desperate need for abortions from Hotline callers, Linda and her colleagues believed there was a simple solution: "I would like to see as many of the blue states as possible embrace telemedicine abortion into the red states by whatever means it takes to make that legal." What Linda envisioned is for abortion-supportive states to change their laws so that licensed providers in those states do not violate that state's laws by mailing pills to other states, even if the provider isn't licensed there and even if abortion is against the law there. Linda understands that there is nothing an abortion-supportive state can do to change the laws of a state where abortion is banned. But Linda wouldn't be physically located in those states, nor would she have a license in those states. Rather, she would have her New York license, be physically located in New York, and—if

New York passed a law like what Linda is envisioning—would not be violating New York law. As part of the law protecting providers like Linda, New York wouldn't cooperate with any other state trying to take legal action—whether criminal or civil—against Linda.

Changing a state's law like this would significantly expand abortion pill access in the country post-*Dobbs*. The American organizations that were mailing or delivering pills to patients in the immediate aftermath of *Dobbs*, such as Abortion On Demand or Just The Pill, were doing so only in states where they are licensed and abortion remains legal. The model Linda envisioned goes further and proposes to provide care to patients in states where abortion is banned. This would once again make provider-supported abortion care available to everyone in the country, something that hasn't existed since the day *Dobbs* was decided.

Linda stressed to us that she understands there are risks with this approach. Under traditional conceptions of health law, states consider care to be rendered where the patient is located, not where the provider is located. Thus, the states where patients receive and use the pills that Linda provides them would view her and anyone following her lead as criminals. However, Linda is willing to take that risk because the legislation she and other advocates pushed New York and other states to pass would prevent her from being extradited and would stop New York court, law enforcement, and administrative officials from cooperating with out-of-state legal actions in most ways. The law would also protect her New York medical license and malpractice insurance.

Linda knows that this protection exists only if she stays in New York. She told us she has been advised not to travel to any of the states with bans because of the possibility of being arrested for violating abortion bans in the state where her patients live, and she was OK with that. "You know, I'm seventy," she said to us. "If I am banned from twenty-six states in the US, that's OK. I can live with that."

When we talked with Linda in 2022, she was in the middle of lobbying the New York legislature and governor's office to change that state's laws. She and her colleagues were unsuccessful in 2022, but ultimately prevailed in 2023.* Many states had passed general shield laws that protect abortion

---

*Full disclosure: One of the authors of this book, David, worked with Linda and other providers and advocates on this effort in 2022 and 2023, as well as on similar efforts in other states.

providers from out-of-state interference, but most states did not include within those laws protection for telehealth provision into states with abortion bans. In 2022, soon after we talked with Linda about her frustrations in New York, Massachusetts passed the first shield law that includes this extra protection, known as a telehealth shield law. Washington, Colorado, Vermont, New York, and California followed in 2023, and Maine joined the list in 2024.

New York's law paved the way for Linda and several of her colleagues in these states to start doing exactly what she told us she would do in 2022. Within weeks of the passage of the New York law, media reports indicated that American telehealth shield providers, as they have become known, mailed over 3,500 doses of abortion pills to patients in states with abortion bans; that number almost doubled by the start of 2024.[10] Linda and her colleagues worked with Aid Access, an overseas abortion provider who previously had been sending pills from India to states with bans and taking two to three weeks to do so. Now, with American providers mailing the pills, patients receive them within days.

Linda has been featured prominently in the press about this new service delivery model. So far, antiabortion advocates and politicians have grumbled about these laws but there have yet to be any legal repercussions, but it's possible that could change at any time, and the telehealth shield laws could be tested. Until then, providers like Linda who are using these telehealth shield laws to send pills to people in states with bans are helping expand access for thousands of patients every month, patients who might otherwise have been unable to access abortion because of post-*Dobbs* state abortion bans.

AN ONLINE INFORMATION HUB

Of course, in order to benefit from these expanded access models, people need to know about medication abortion and how to access it. If they don't, all of the developments in service delivery already described as well as the other novel approaches being taken in response to *Dobbs* would be useless because no one would know about them. In the wake of *Dobbs*, many people in the abortion rights and justice movement understand the urgency of getting information out to the public now that *Roe* has been overruled and are working to do so.

Francine Coeytaux is what you might call an abortion pill proselytizer. One of the cofounders and codirectors of Plan C, Francine believes that, were it not for restrictions on distribution, a much higher percentage of people in the United States who want an abortion would use abortion pills. When we first talked with her pre-*Dobbs*, she pointed us to countries in Europe, such as Finland and Sweden, where more than 95 percent of abortions are by abortion pills. She certainly doesn't want to force a method of abortion on anyone and is a strong believer in personal choice. However, she thinks that too many providers in the United States have a bias against abortion pills. Her mission is to change the narrative of abortion in this country so that abortion pills are much more common, especially post-*Dobbs*.

What makes Francine such a believer is her conviction that abortion pills offer access without gatekeepers and put control more directly in the hands of the users. As Francine and many others see it, there is no need to involve someone trained in medicine in dispensing them. Requiring this is what she calls "medicalization," and she complained that "medicalization of these pills is so deep." However, as Francine repeatedly told us, it doesn't have to be this way because the pills are safe and easy to use. Laws requiring medical doctors to be gatekeepers are typically used to control providers. If people don't need medical expertise to control when and how they can get pills, it will be harder to use the legal system to stop access to pills. Francine's vision is that "pills should be in the hands of people who want to use them."

Francine has the long experience in reproductive health service delivery to push toward that reality today. She started her journey as a reproductive health advocate in the 1970s, when she was a student and spent a year abroad in Peru. There, she was assigned to conduct interviews with women coming to a low-income pediatric clinic. Over and over from the women she talked with she heard "Help me not have another child." That experience led her to dedicate her life to family planning and finding ways to give people control over their reproduction. Her first jobs after college were with Planned Parenthood in San Francisco, conducting teen outreach, and then with the California Department of Education, working in migrant education.

After getting a graduate degree in public health, Francine worked for the Population Council in sub-Saharan Africa, where she helped introduce new reproductive technologies, including Norplant (the first implantable contraceptive), emergency contraceptives (such as Plan B), and, ultimately, abortion pills (mifepristone and misoprostol). By the 2000s, she said, "the rest of the world had moved to abortion pills and the US had their head in the sand and most didn't even know what these pills were." She was learning about models such as Women on Web that mailed pills to women who didn't want to be pregnant anymore so that they could "totally self-manage their abortions, without going to doctors."

The goal that she and her cofounders, Amy Merrill and Elisa Wells, had when they started Plan C in 2015 was to bring the United States into alignment with modern abortion practice. As the Plan C website states on its "About Us" page, the organization "transforms access to abortion in the US by normalizing the self-directed option of abortion pills by mail." The organization envisions "a near future in which the ability to end an early pregnancy is directly in the hands of anyone who seeks it." Once *Roe* was overturned, Francine felt that this mission and vision took on even greater importance.

Plan C's greatest visibility is its website, a comprehensive online hub for information about abortion pills. It has pages about abortion pill basics such as how to use them and what their safety record is. It also has information about pill-related legal issues and sources of medical and emotional support for those who use the pills. Possibly the most important part of the Plan C website is the "Find Pills" drop-down menu on the home page that opens up to a list of all states and territories, including those with bans and restricted access. Users input the state or territory where they are located then find all of the options available to them for accessing abortion pills where they live. For states where abortion is not banned, Plan C has three categories of options: US-based telehealth services, websites that sell pills, and in-person clinics in or near the state. The first two options do not require going to an in-person clinic and are entirely online or by phone; the difference is that the telehealth services involve interaction with a medical care provider before obtaining pills and often days or weeks after taking the pills while the websites that sell pills at very low cost (some for as low as $36) do so directly to the patient without provider involvement. The third category lists two different websites that help people find the closest brick-and-mortar clinics that provide abortion pills to patients, whether in-state or by traveling.

States where abortion is banned show a fourth option, community networks. These are volunteer groups of lay individuals who work under the radar to ship or deliver pills for free directly to people who need them. These pills tend to be generic versions of abortion drugs that volunteers mail or deliver directly to people who need them. These networks must operate with extreme care because of state antiabortion laws, but they are committed to making sure that as many people as possible can obtain pills, even if they live in states that ban abortion.

A key point, Francine explained, is that every service listed on Plan C has been vetted by the organization so that people visiting the website can be confident they are obtaining accurate and safe information. The vetting process involves testing websites and providers by purchasing pills to verify that the pills that are shipped are actually mifepristone and misoprostol. However, users are warned that just because the services listed were reliable in the past does not guarantee they will be in the future.

The goal of the Plan C website is to make sure people have all the needed information about how to obtain pills, how to use them, and how to manage their abortion safely. "We're trying to get people more information than just where do you get the product," Francine told us. The site also prominently features the Miscarriage and Abortion Hotline, the hotline Linda Prine helped start that is staffed by medical professionals to help people who have medical questions about using pills. That way, if people who have obtained pills without the help of a clinician (from websites that sell pills or community networks) have medical questions related to the use of the pills, they have a place to turn to get answers.

As Francine tells it, the three biggest challenges for Plan C since the overturning of *Roe* have been increasing awareness about the option of mailed pills, keeping on top of changes in the landscape including legal issues, and fighting stigma and fear. After Texas implemented SB8 in late 2021, the site saw an increased number of visitors from Texas. But once *Dobbs* was decided, the increase was nationwide, and the spike continued through the end of 2022. She told us Plan C has evidence that the site is "at the crossroads of information, directing traffic to information about anything that has to do with abortion pills online." To get the word out, Plan C has been using online ads targeting specific states as well as billboards and signs in specific localities. All of this directs people to Plan C to find vetted information about how to find pills.

Plan C's task of assessing the accuracy of the information it provides also became more difficult after *Dobbs*. Before *Dobbs*, when abortion was legal in every state, there were fewer informal networks and web-based pharmacies for the organization to vet. But now, Francine said, with more people jumping on the opportunity to provide abortion pills, "We can barely stay on top of them, they're popping up so often." But doing so is an essential part of the site's mission, so they prioritize staying up-to-date to make sure the providers and sellers are legitimate and the changes are accurately reflected on the site.

Doing all of this in the new legal environment has made Plan C a target. Francine told us that she and her colleagues have been watching the anti-abortion movement's messaging around pills and what they say about Plan C in particular. "We monitor it quite closely because we're trying to understand how they see us," she said. "In the antiabortion literature, Plan C is at the very top of what they think is evil and breaking all the rules."

This attention highlights the importance of understanding and preparing for possible legal conflict. By the end of 2022, Francine told us, Plan C had an agreement with lawyers to work with them on health law and First Amendment issues, but she indicated that the attorneys were there to help if any issues arose, not to give advice to Plan C about how to change its model because of legal concerns. "Our role with Plan C is to share information, and we know we have a First Amendment right to do that. And we think that, should we be attacked, we would not be found liable," she told us, referring to the possibility of being sued for aiding in an illegal abortion. "We know we're evidence-based and just sharing information, and we are not going to be told that we can't do this." She worried that a lot of organizations in the movement have been "retrenching" and "stepping back" out of fear of legal repercussions, but Plan C is "stepping up" its work. It angers Francine that providers and patients are going to be criminalized because of pills, so she wants Plan C to be there for them "to give them the support and the resources of whom to turn to and what to know, and how to protect, and how to defend against possible criminalization."

This commitment to getting information to people who need it without backing down infuses another key aspect of Plan C's mission, one that has increased in importance since *Dobbs*. Francine said that an essential part of what Plan C does is "catalyzing action for anybody willing to just kind of push the envelope." Plan C has supported efforts to obtain missed-period pills, pills prescribed or obtained without verifying first if someone is pregnant. If the person is pregnant, the pills will end the pregnancy, as they are the same pills used for an abortion. The organization also supports advanced provision of abortion pills, to be used sometime in the future if the need arises, like people buying Advil before they have a headache. Plan C also makes grants to other entities, such as those experimenting with telehealth provision of care, so they can develop novel models of care that expand access. And Plan C supports and provides information about patients using a service to forward mailed abortion pills from a state where abortion is legal into a state where abortion is illegal, something that some people see as too risky.

Francine understands that Plan C's support of all of these various approaches to putting pills in the hands of those who need them worries some lawyers and others concerned with legal ramifications. But she and her colleagues are standing firm. Francine stressed again that what Plan C is doing is just providing information, and she firmly believes that this is not a legal problem. "The people who are taking the risk are the people who are [taking the pills], but we're definitely going to let people know that these systems work." Although so far nothing has happened, with a target on Plan C's back, Francine said, "If we're a test case, we're prepared."

SPREADING THE WORD, CHANGING THE CULTURE

Whereas Plan C focuses on the specifics of how to obtain and use abortion pills, others are focusing on the more general goal of informing the public about abortion pills. Amelia Bonow, the cofounder and director of Shout Your Abortion, told us that "the best thing that you can do right now to help us expand abortion access is to spread the word about abortion pills."

Amelia started the organization in 2015 after her experience telling her abortion story online. Amelia had been living in Seattle, bartending to work her way through graduate school. She had studied issues related to abortion as an undergraduate student while majoring in cultural anthropology, and previously volunteered at Planned Parenthood, so was already committed to issues of reproductive justice.

In September of that year, in response to congressional attacks on Planned Parenthood, Amelia posted on Facebook that she had had an abortion the year before. Amelia described her experience, unlike many narratives about abortion in the popular press, in very positive terms, writing that she remembered the experience "with a nearly inexpressible level of gratitude" and received "exceptional" care. She said that too much of the political discourse is based on "the assumption that abortion is still something to be whispered about" and that abortion should be accompanied by "some level of sadness, shame, or regret." But Amelia didn't feel that way. She ended her post, "I have a good heart and having an abortion made me happy in a totally unqualified way. Why wouldn't I be happy that I was not forced to become a mother. #ShoutYourAbortion"[11]

Amelia's post went viral. Some of her friends re-posted it, including one who was a well-known media commentator, and people all over the country began posting their own abortion stories. Within days the hashtag #ShoutYourAbortion had been used over 200,000 times. Amelia became a media sensation, giving countless interviews about the importance of busting abortion stigma and people speaking openly about their abortions. She also received intense backlash and threats, resulting at one point in her leaving her home to go into hiding.[12]

The upside of the experience was that Amelia quit her job and her graduate program and started the organization Shout Your Abortion, SYA for short. From the beginning, SYA's mission has been to destigmatize abortion by creating platforms for people to share their stories and by using art and creativity to push for the normalization of abortion in the culture at large.

More recently, SYA has also focused on informing the public about, as Amelia phrased it, "safe paths to access, regardless of legality." This focus was inspired in part by Amelia visiting Poland to connect with activists there that SYA had been working in tandem with for a number of years. Amelia observed activists in Poland working to put together a network to support abortion seekers and to help them access pills despite the fact that abortion has been illegal in the country for decades. Amelia saw firsthand the importance of having fearless voices informing the public about safe abortion methods and practical avenues to access them.

With the Supreme Court decision about the fate of *Roe* looming, Amelia told us in the beginning of 2022 about SYA's focus on getting information to the public about abortion pills. "The landscape has changed," she said. "There are now many sources of abortion pills that are activist vetted and medically safe, and people need to know that this option exists." She called dispensing information about pills "low-hanging fruit when it comes to expanding abortion access" and "a new front in activism."

Amelia sees SYA's work in an era without *Roe* as complementing Plan C's. She called that website's information "granular" in terms of finding out exactly how to access and use pills and then get medical and legal information if needed. "If I'm actually a person looking for pills, where do I get that information? Plan C feels like that place to me." What SYA does on top of that is act as a "top-level megaphone that is saying, 'Hey, everyone, this exists.'"

The way SYA accomplishes this goal is different than how Plan C functions as a centralized source of information. Amelia emphasized, in response to *Dobbs*, that the most important message she and SYA can convey is one of defiance. SYA is modeling its abortion pill campaigns on those of ACT-UP, the organization started in the 1980s to bring direct action to the fight against AIDS. "ACT-UP has been incredibly influential to me," Amelia told us. "I think that in terms of the material wins that they achieved and also of the culture change that they achieved in a very short time, they are an unparalleled model of successful activism."

Amelia told us about several different plans to inform the public about pills. In December 2021, the day the Supreme Court heard oral argument in *Dobbs*, Amelia and three other SYA activists stood on the steps of the Supreme Court and swallowed abortion pills, even though they weren't pregnant. Behind them was a banner that read, "We Are Taking Abortion Pills Forever." The direct action attracted much media attention, helping spread the word about pills.[13]

After *Dobbs*, there were other tactics—even street actions. She and her colleagues trained local community groups how to get the word out about pills in the communities where they live. They've hired a billboard truck to drive through areas where abortion is banned with information about pills and how to get them. They set up "lemonade stands" that gave out boxes labeled as abortion pills, though with information inside rather than actual pills; these "lemonade stands" have been replicated by activists all over the country approximately fifty times. SYA distributed signs using abortion pills to form letters that spelled out "I will aid and abet abortion." Amelia has even contemplated mass pill taking at state capitals in states with abortion bans and using a catapult to send abortion pills across state lines from states where abortion is legal into states where it is banned.

Perhaps the highest-profile event for Amelia was when she appeared on stage at the December 2022 People's Choice Awards as a guest of the pop star Lizzo, who invited seventeen activists in all different fields on stage with her. She chose Amelia because of SYA's work in a year when abortion lost its status as a constitutional right. Amelia was incredibly grateful for the opportunity to be surrounded by such dynamic activists. "We spent a lot of time just surrounding these women with love and really bonding with each other."

In her spirit of defiance, Amelia didn't miss her opportunity to get her message across. "They told us, 'No words on stage,' and I just, obviously, did it anyway." When she was introduced by Lizzo as someone working to "increase awareness of abortion pills" and again, at the end in the group gathering, Amelia smiled and held up a sign that said "Abortion Pills Forever." She joked with us, "I'm like, 'What? Are you going to be mad that I did an activism? That's on you.'"

Amelia's ultimate goal for SYA in the age of *Dobbs* is to support an "intentionally diffuse cultural movement" of people informing others about abortion pills and ways to obtain them, especially for people in states with abortion bans. How that happens needs to be, as she explained, "locally determined because the landscapes are so specific." In getting this information out about pills, Amelia hopes to normalize them as an option for everyone, no matter the state, whether with medical professional assistance or not, whether through legal means or informal community networks that operate outside the boundaries of law. Amelia stressed to us that "pills were not a solution in and of themselves but an important part of a larger ecosystem of access." Accordingly, SYA also trains activists to support local abortion funds and independent clinics.

When information about pills proliferates, Amelia said, there is an opportunity post-*Dobbs*: "We have the tools to create a meaningful landscape of abortion access in post-*Dobbs* America, but we need to dramatically increase the level of participation. We need people to stop seeing abortion as something that they can only have if a court gives them the right to it and start seeing access as something which fundamentally belongs to all of us, which is ours, currently and definitively, and which we can have to the degree that we work to facilitate it in our communities."

TRANSFORMING ABORTION PROVISION

It will be years before we have complete data about the impact of abortion pills on the post-*Dobbs* landscape. The #WeCount study has captured the increase in virtual clinics providing pills in the nine months after *Dobbs*. In that time frame, the study found an 85 percent increase in abortions provided by virtual-only providers over the pre-*Dobbs* months. Immediately before *Dobbs*, there were on average 4,025 abortions per month from virtual-only providers; after *Dobbs*, the monthly average was 7,461 abortions.[14] These numbers are certainly undercounts, as the study looks only at provision of pills within the formal healthcare system.

The people profiled in this chapter, and others working toward the same goals, are a big part of this post-*Dobbs* story. With everything these people have been doing to increase access to and promote abortion pills—within established medical protocols, pushing their limits, and beyond—it seems that *Dobbs*, paradoxically, has propelled the abortion landscape to offer more options than ever existed before.

Francine Coeytaux suggested as much to us. "I believe we in the US are getting in a progressively better position," she said. "I do believe there is better access these days." It will take a longer period of time before we know if that's true, but if it is, it'll be because there are many people like Linda Prine, who told us that abortion pills enable people like her "to figure out all the workarounds we can," and others, like Amelia Bonow, who believe that abortion pills mean "you cannot stop this" because they empower people to say "fuck these courts, we're doing it anyway."

CHAPTER SEVEN

SUPPORTING PATIENTS

Switchboard, boom, boom, boom, boom, boom. I
think we calculated it. It ended up being around a
250 percent increase in our calls almost immediately.

—CHLOE HANSON HEBERT,
National Abortion Hotline

Even before *Dobbs*, when abortion was legal in every state, it was far from easily accessible for everyone. Our previous book, *Obstacle Course*, chronicled all the ways that states created obstacles to people obtaining an abortion, from burdensome counseling requirements to unnecessary waiting periods to arbitrary gestational limits and more.[1] Two of the most consequential barriers people faced were traveling long distances to a clinic and paying for the abortion.

In the period when *Roe* was the law of the land, abortion clinics were often located in densely populated areas, and some states had only one clinic. People looking to get to a clinic frequently faced lengthy trips. Compounding the problem was the reality that roughly three-quarters of abortion patients live in poverty. For many who sought abortions the expenses of travel were prohibitive.

Even if patients could afford to travel to a clinic, they still had to pay for the abortion. Compared to other medical care in the United States, abortion isn't that expensive, costing roughly six or seven hundred dollars in the first trimester and rising to a couple thousand dollars later in the second trimester. However, for those living close to or at the poverty line, that is a lot of money. Normally, Medicaid would cover healthcare for people who are struggling, but because of the federal Hyde Amendment and state versions that accomplish the same goal, in most states, Medicaid is prohibited from covering all but the most exceptional abortions.[2]

Volunteer networks of drivers and nonprofit organizations that paid for some of the cost of abortions helped many people, but these practical obstacles made it difficult for many people to access care. And that was before *Dobbs*.

Now that *Dobbs* is the law of the land, these access problems have become even more daunting. With abortion illegal in fourteen states and highly restricted in several others, travel times have grown exponentially for people who want to get to the closest state that has an open abortion clinic.

Caitlin Myers is an economics professor who has long tracked abortion travel. In the year following *Dobbs*, she found that the average travel distance to get to an abortion provider jumped from twenty-five to eighty-six miles, almost 3.5 times more. The percentage of people in the United States living more than two hundred miles from an abortion provider went from 1 percent to 14 percent of the population. If the antiabortion movement's attacks on abortion pills were ever successful in removing them from the market, these travel distances would skyrocket, as many of the roughly 40 percent of abortion clinics that are medication-only clinics would stop offering abortion services.[3]

Traveling to get an abortion complicates everything. It requires time—not just for the travel itself, but for the planning, for staying overnight wherever you travel to, and for any hiccups along the way. The average one-way travel time to a clinic in a state where abortion is legal for someone living in Texas or Louisiana is now seven hours. The round trip could take multiple days and incur myriad expenses. That amount of time requires being able to take time off work and family obligations, such as caring for children or other loved ones.

Travel also requires safety. People whom government officials might suspect of being unlawfully in this country risk being stopped and detained at government checkpoints or airports, and people of color risk being stopped by police on highways. Travel also requires familiarity. For many people, managing the interstate highway system or navigating airports is second nature, but for those who have not had the privilege of traveling regularly in their lives, all of this can be difficult to navigate.

But probably most difficult, travel requires money. Everything about travel costs money, regardless of the mode of travel: gas money, car upkeep, airfare, food, hotel, childcare, taxis, and more. It all adds up, and that's on top of the cost of the abortion, which, because travel comes with delays, can be more expensive because the price of an abortion increases as someone progresses later into pregnancy. Before *Dobbs*, these costs were high for many and prohibitive for some. Post *Dobbs*, everything is more expensive.[4]

One of this book's authors, David, has been working to assist patients with transportation, practical support, and funding for decades. When he left his full-time practice as an attorney and started in academia, one of the first things he did was contact his local abortion fund to see if he could help in any way, and he served on their board for six years. After that he worked with other people interested in reproductive rights and justice to start a practical support group for the Philadelphia area in 2016. Since then he has been a regular driver and one of a rotating cadre of weekly coordinators who help arrange travel and overnight stays for abortion patients in the region, ranging from ten-minute drives to multiday travel plans.

The effect of *Dobbs* on his work was evident, even in an area of the country without abortion bans. Patients from states with bans now travel to the Philadelphia area in higher numbers than before *Dobbs*. The numbers are not astronomical, as the Philadelphia region is not the closest area to any state with a ban, but even an additional one or two patients a week needing assistance because they are traveling from long distances consume enormous resources.

The people profiled in this chapter have been tackling the formidable task of funding and supporting patients for years. In 2022 and 2023, they saw a complete shift in the landscape for abortion access and rushed to fill the need. Working with local nonprofits and loosely knit groups of volunteers, they moved from a model that, for the most part, had supported patients traveling *within* a state to a model of supporting patients traveling *among* states. This required a rethinking of travel logistics as well as a dramatic increase in financial support—which so far they've been fortunate to receive.

But a lot about this new environment remains a mystery. There is no way to know just how many people have slipped through the cracks and not been able to get a sought-after abortion. And there is certainly no way of predicting what has been one of the biggest questions on many people's minds: whether the "rage donations" that have funded almost all of their post-*Dobbs* work will continue into the future. Because if that were to change and donations were to drop off, all the heroic efforts described in this chapter that have enabled people to continue to obtain abortions post-*Dobbs*, and maybe even all of the efforts described in this book, would be seriously threatened.

LOCAL AND REGIONAL SUPPORT

The big question, as Oriaku Njoku (who uses she/they pronouns, so here we will use both interchangeably) sees it, the question that she talks with so many others about in the wake of *Dobbs*, is "How far are you willing to go for our collective liberation?" Because to Oriaku, for people supporting abortion patients, now that there is no national right to abortion, the risks and threats are everywhere. The work that Oriaku has been doing for almost a decade to help patients get to abortion appointments has taken on new dimensions that they were prepared for in theory but now have to meet in reality. Everything Oriaku does is infused with notions of racial and reproductive justice, so she knows that the risks for Black people, like her, are different: "The reality is that white people driving through the middle of a rural city at the end of the night is going to look different than me driving through the rural city in the middle of the night."

This fine attention to the promise of collective resistance in a world of racial and reproductive injustice has been at the heart of Oriaku's work in the movement. They had just finished working a retail job at the end of 2012 when a friend brought Oriaku to a training in reproductive justice. At the time, Oriaku's main interest was in immigration reform. The training Oriaku attended connected immigration to reproductive justice and, for the first time, exposed her to a broad intersectional framework.

After attending a reproductive justice conference in 2013, she was hooked. "It was at that moment that I was like, 'Oh my goodness. Being Black, first-generation Nigerian American, queer, fat, Southern—all of these things—there's a place for all of that within the movement. I don't have to silo my life. I don't have to compartmentalize things.' I thought, 'I have to do something.' To be my whole self consistently, that is something I want. And I want everyone to have that."

It all started on the phones. Oriaku was working the front-desk phones at a massage business when she saw an opening at one of the local Atlanta abortion clinics for a phone advocate, and she leapt at the opportunity to take her phone skills and use them in abortion movement work. It was in doing that work, talking with people on the phone about how to make ends meet to get an abortion, that Oriaku realized her calling in abortion funding and practical support.

She explained her epiphany to us. "We've got to do something. This is a mess. There are too many times where we talk to someone whose escort decided to bail on them or they couldn't find childcare or they've been waiting weeks to raise five hundred dollars only to find out that, now that they're sixteen weeks, it is double the amount. So I was like, 'We can start a fund. And not only a fund, but we can start an organization organizing around this. Because this is not what it should be.'"

From that spark, Oriaku and others working alongside her started ARC-Southeast (ARC stands for Access Reproductive Care), a reproductive-justice organization providing abortion funding and practical support to Southerners. At first, Oriaku continued working at Atlanta clinics, but then left that work to work full-time for ARC-Southeast. Oriaku attributes their willingness to shake things up and create a new organization to their being new to the movement. They told us, "Having done work outside of the movement, knowing the world we live in and not thinking just in the movement, I'm always critical. It doesn't have to be like this. We have power, and we can change this stuff."

When we first talked with Oriaku in early 2022, in her role as the executive director for ARC-Southeast, she was engaged in a two-part struggle: helping Southerners, including those in Texas dealing with SB8, and scenario planning for the possible end of *Roe* later that year. In some ways, Oriaku explained to us, the SB8 work along with the difficult access issues people already faced in the South was actually part of the scenario planning. "We know," they said. "We've been living in the South. We've been living under these conditions for decades. What's new is that it's going to be more difficult to navigate a lot of the already-hard obstacles that it takes to currently get an abortion in the South."

In early 2022, the difficulties SB8 was causing for people across the South were front of Oriaku's mind. ARC-Southeast was helping Texans travel to Mississippi, Alabama, Georgia, even Florida to get care. This displacement caused ripple effects that affected other people ARC-Southeast helped. As Texans flooded these other Southern states, wait times increased for everyone, sometimes causing local patients to have to travel to other states or even other regions of the country to get timely care. ARC-Southeast assisted callers with every part of this challenge, from planning to travel to funding. ARC-Southeast provided volunteer drivers, bus fare, hotel rooms, direct transfer of funds, and increased funding for abortions. In all of this, Oriaku explained, it's a "collaborative effort" with the caller. "We're never, like, 'We're going to do this *for* you.' It's like, 'We're going to do this *with* you.'"

All the SB8 work helped ARC-Southeast plan for *Dobbs*. The organization committed itself to finding volunteers to drive across state lines and to funding people as much as they could. Oriaku told us that she understood the legal risk involved for ARC-Southeast and its staff but that she was having conversations with staff and volunteers about everyone's risk tolerance and then planning on how to assist anyone who might be arrested. "The reality is," it seemed to Oriaku in 2022, "folks are going to be criminalized, and we want to make sure that we're protecting the folks doing the work as well."

Once *Roe* was overturned, the challenges ARC-Southeast had been experiencing because of SB8 and planning for beyond Texas came to the fore. "It was wild," Oriaku told us. Immediately after *Dobbs*, Mississippi, Alabama, and Tennessee banned abortion, so ARC-Southeast had to quickly pivot and coordinate even more patient travel to Georgia and Florida. Then Georgia implemented its six-week ban in late July (as discussed in chapter 4). ARC-Southeast had to refocus its efforts once again, continuing to support patients going to Florida but now working with patients to get to South Carolina and North Carolina as well. Everyone at ARC-Southeast kept their eyes on the same goal: "Let's help you get where you need to go." The grand scale of coordination made Oriaku reflect, "It feels like we're a travel agency."

Soon after *Dobbs*, Oriaku transitioned to a new job that would allow them to take their experience with ARC-Southeast and use it to benefit local abortion funds around the country. In mid-July, they accepted a position as the executive director of the National Network of Abortion Funds (NNAF). Oriaku continues to live in Atlanta and remains connected to ARC-Southeast but described the transition to a different organization as "bittersweet. We all cried."

In this new role, Oriaku leads an organization that has one hundred members that are all local abortion funds—these funds raise money to help pay for the various costs associated with abortion care, and some also provide practical support to abortion patients, for example, help with arranging air travel and lodging. NNAF does not itself directly fund abortion;

with its large staff and thousands of individual donors, it provides extensive assistance to local practical support and funding organizations through grants, leadership development, infrastructure support, and technical assistance. Oriaku is committed to this new work because she believes that helping build the infrastructure of abortion networks and funds around the country is how more people can access care post-*Dobbs*.

The new numbers of abortion seekers crossing state lines means that funds that assist patients in states with bans have to build connections with clinics in a variety of places where abortion remains legal because traveling patients will need options. Thinking back to their time at ARC-Southeast, Oriaku explained that travel is more complicated than people assume, and patients may end up traveling to places much farther away than the closest open clinics.

Oriaku drew on the migration patterns of Black people during the Great Migration from the South to the North that started in the early twentieth century. For instance, many Black people from the South migrated to Chicago, so some patients may drive to Chicago, where they have family and friends, rather than going to unfamiliar places in southern Illinois. Furthermore, Oriaku pointed out, there are still plenty of places in the country where Black people don't feel safe. "I'm just imagining why would you think that it is OK to have folks from the South travel through 'sundown cities,'" she said, referring to locations where Black people have historically been terrorized once night fell.[5] "It's not making sense."

Navigating different cultures is another challenge for many Southerners seeking abortion. Oriaku described one of the overlooked difficulties with this kind of travel for care—the need for "culturally competent care." She talked about the culture shock that some Southerners have going to big Northern cities like New York for care. It's not uncommon for travelers leaving a state with an abortion ban to be in a big city for the first time. Everyone involved, from the helpers to the funders to the clinic staff, needs to understand, Oriaku said, "that we don't know what they went through to get here, to get to the clinic, to get to the appointment."

It's important, she continued, to know that "an abortion is just a moment in these people's lives" and to "think about the person and not just the patient." With so many people traveling to places outside their comfort zone, Oriaku was concerned that this nuance would be lost and patients would be treated more transactionally and less as the whole people they are.

One of the recurring issues with practical support that Oriaku hopes to tackle in their new national role is streamlining the process for patients. Oriaku and others in the movement envision working toward a system in which a patient would be able to make one phone call to get their appointment, funding, support, and any other needs met. Such a system would eliminate what Oriaku called "the hustle and hassle" that abortion patients frequently experience coordinating everything that it takes to get care. Developing this system will take a lot of work, but Oriaku is committed to national infrastructure improvements like this to make it easier for patients, especially those with increased needs post-*Dobbs*, and hopes to use their leadership position to nudge the movement in this direction.

Working as she does with so many groups around the country, Oriaku has a bird's-eye view of the challenges the staff of abortion funds face in the new post-*Roe* environment. Chief among these challenges has been managing risk. With abortion illegal in so many states, can abortion funds help people in those states obtain an abortion in other states where abortion remains legal? NNAF has legal assistance to help it and its staff work through these issues, and many local funds do as well. Although she is personally "down to do all the wild things," Oriaku knows it is different for institutions and other individuals making their own personal risk assessments.

NNAF is not "telling folks or making suggestions to funds, as far as what to do," Oriaku told us, but rather is helping them think through realities, risks, and opportunities. People must also, importantly, trust that any decision a fund makes with respect to its own risks is the right decision for that fund, whether it's a risk-tolerant decision to continue helping patients despite legal threats or a risk-averse decision to pause funding or assistance in the face of the new environment. Oriaku explained as an example, what if a fund has an employee who is undocumented? Only that fund in conjunction with that employee can truly assess the risk the employee might face if any legal threat materialized.

One of the other challenges abortion-fund staff have faced post-*Dobbs* is dealing with growth, in numbers of both paid staff and volunteers. NNAF itself has grown in the wake of the decision, as have local funds. This means training new employees and making sure the organization has the necessary infrastructure. *Dobbs* has also meant more people reaching out to NNAF and its member organizations to volunteer. Oriaku drew on her experience with ARC-Southeast, when SB8 and increasingly hostile restrictions on abortions in the Southeast led to the organization being swamped with new volunteer applications. Having more people to help with funding and practical support is, of course, a good thing, but Oriaku stressed that it is important that new folks be informed, vetted, and trained, all of which takes time and resources.

But the growth also presented new opportunities, as the new volunteers often bring a wide diversity of skills to organizations. Oriaku said, "We noticed that volunteers are wanting to do other things, as well, to support the work that is going on." When people inquire what they can do, Oriaku encourages them to think, "What brings you joy? What are you good at? What's the skill that you have?" Whether it's graphic design or flying a plane or doing administrative work, abortion funds can usually find some way to use those skills, given the difficult road in front of them. It all leads back to funding more support and more abortions, because, as Oriaku explained, if a volunteer is doing the administrative work, "it increases the capacity of the fund to do more of that abortion-funding work."

In her new role in this new environment, Oriaku sees opportunity in building and leveraging cultural capital. "I'm excited I have this national platform," Oriaku told us. She intends to "shake some stuff up" by taking advantage of the post-*Dobbs* attention on abortion to talk about abortion in new ways with new audiences and focus them on the importance of helping patients obtain access. She was excited about celebrities who were not just talking about helping Planned Parenthood, the almost-reflexive response many people have when thinking about supporting abortion, but were instead talking about supporting NNAF and local abortion funds. She was particularly excited about the pop star Lizzo using her platform to say she was donating money to NNAF. "People are starting to understand what abortion funds do, how they show up, and how powerful we are," Oriaku said.

Under *Roe*, for a long time people took abortion for granted and ignored the access challenges that had been bubbling under the surface, Oriaku said. But now, with *Roe* overturned, people are scrambling to figure out what to do. Referring to organizations like ARC-Southeast and NNAF, Oriaku said, "We saw this parade coming down Main Street. We knew this was happening. We felt it. There's two ways we can go about it now. We can say, 'We've been telling y'all.' Or, we can say, 'OK, join us.

We are now ready, and we've been waiting for you, so let's figure out how to do this work together.'" Oriaku is committed to the latter approach through outreach, visibility, organizing, political education, and cultivating new connections and donors.

With this national attention on abortion, Oriaku's work is to translate it into real improvements in access. It's not enough, they explained, to fund politicians and legal advocacy. Patient support and access need real investment too. "If we have all this cultural capital that we're harnessing, but the foundations and donors are either hesitant or feel out of touch with what the need actually is on the ground, that is something that gives me a lot of pause. A lot of this could look really different if they divested from some organizations and invested in some of the groups who are actually on the ground doing the work." Making sure that the spike in donations and investments goes to abortion funds who make abortion a reality for people who need one is an essential part of this new role for Oriaku.

Looking more broadly, Oriaku sees great possibilities in mobilizing the fund community, especially in regions of the country where abortion is banned. That requires connecting the threats to reproductive freedom to other forms of oppression and the country's increasingly conservative politics. Reflecting on her time at ARC-Southeast, Oriaku told us she was always excited about politicizing the people ARC-Southeast helps by encouraging them, after they received care and once they're safe and comfortable, to share their story. Or even, when the people ARC-Southeast worked with are able, to volunteer, donate, or fundraise for ARC-Southeast. Oriaku wants funds to create "that brave space of community of folks who have had abortions to continue to talk about their experiences." In communicating in real language about their situations, people can, Oriaku shared, "build power" and "mobilize folks."

As Oriaku looks to the future, she knows that people ask why she hasn't moved to a more abortion-friendly place because of the work she does. But Oriaku is defiantly remaining in Atlanta. "How are we going to create the change that we want if all of us move to New York?" she asked us. "I'm choosing to stay with my people." At the end of the day, Oriaku's defiance is mixed with a healthy dose of determined optimism. "I don't like losing, and I play to win," she declared. Ultimately, she concluded, about herself, ARC-Southeast, NNAF, and local funds more generally, "We're doing this, no matter what."

NATIONAL SUPPORT

For weeks, Chloe Hanson Hebert and Rachel Lachenauer had been waiting anxiously. Like everyone in the abortion world, they had read the
leaked *Dobbs* opinion in early May 2022 and knew what was coming. They
knew that this would mean a flood of callers for the National Abortion
Hotline, a resource created by the National Abortion Federation (NAF),
where they both were directors. They, like everyone else, didn't know the
precise day the Hotline would be inundated. "For weeks," Rachel said,
"we'd been playing this horrible, no good, very bad game of watching the
Supreme Court blog at ten a.m. Everybody was living with such anxiety,
which is really not healthy. But we were all kind of prepared."

The preparation paid off. When the decision came out Friday morning, June 24, the Hotline was ready. "We stayed online through the whole
decision and did not cease operations even for a minute," Chloe recalled.
And the response was almost immediate. Within ten minutes of the decision, "switchboard, boom, boom, boom, boom, boom," Chloe said. "We
calculated it. It ended up being around a 250 percent increase in our calls
almost immediately. It was really incredible."

The *Dobbs* decision's jolt to the Hotline was something Chloe and
Rachel wished they never had to face, even though their decades of experience had prepared them. Chloe's background was in social work,
helping domestic violence and sexual assault survivors. The core of her
work had always been "bodily autonomy and protection," she said. She
had been working for a women's resource center in Arizona when a position with the Hotline became available; in 2022 she was director of
operations. "It felt like the next logical step in terms of bodily autonomy
work for people that are often very marginalized for what they can and
can't do and how that impacts them." When Chloe was hired as a Hotline
director in 2011, it was much smaller than it was in 2022 when *Roe* was
overruled—thirty mostly part-time staff as compared to over fifty full-
time staff in 2022.*

---

*Tragically, Chloe passed away from cancer in April 2023, months after our last in-
terview with her. Her family gave us permission to draw on our interviews with her
for this book. NAF set up a fund in Chloe's memory that helps NAF members who
provide abortion care. "Honoring Our Beloved Colleague Chloe Hanson Hebert,"
National Abortion Federation, https://perma.cc/NNU5-XRCG.

Rachel came to this work from a more specific focus on abortion rights that started early. She was raised in what she called "a New York Jewish liberal household" where "social justice was infused into that culture from a really young age." She went to the March for Women's Lives in 2004 when she was a young teenager and knew that working in abortion rights and access was what she wanted to do with her life. When she was in college in Washington, DC, in 2011, she worked as a part-time Hotline counselor in the evenings. "Then, I just sort of worked my way up from there." Rachel started as a counselor, then became a case manager, and then moved into a director position. When we talked with her in 2022, she was the Hotline's director of patient experience.

Like so many others throughout the abortion world, to prepare for *Dobbs*, Rachel and Chloe drew on their experience handling SB8. Before SB8, the Hotline was well versed in helping patients access appointments and funding in an environment with constantly changing abortion laws. But SB8 was different. "Complying with this law was not just a matter of redirecting patients to available appointments," Rachel said, "but it really forced us to rethink how to provide Hotline services at all"—because of the new legal issues. The Texas law not only drastically cut back on services available to people in Texas, requiring the Hotline to help them find care either within the law in Texas or elsewhere, but it also put patients and helpers at legal risk, forcing the Hotline to think about how to minimize risk to everyone involved, especially its own workers. In a very real way, SB8 was a one-state rehearsal that prepared people for the larger-scale impact of *Dobbs*.

The Hotline made several changes to address SB8. First, it set up a state-specific phone menu option for people calling from Texas so that they could talk directly with Hotline workers who specialized in Texas. Second, the Hotline built up their internal resources to expedite the service they provided to help patients get care within the SB8 six-week cutoff window or, if they couldn't, to help patients travel out of state. Part of that was staffing, and part of that was financial. The staff handling Texas calls prioritized these patients' needs, and the Hotline made more funding available to immediately assist patients with funding in Texas so that funding delays did not push them beyond the cutoff date. "We don't want there to be a financial reason why somebody has to delay that appointment," Rachel explained. "Because by the time they raise even that fifty dollars extra or whatever it might be, their opportunity to be seen anywhere close to home might have evaporated." Third, the Hotline worked with abortion providers in Texas to make sure the process would be coordinated smoothly for the patient while also reducing everybody's legal risk.

Within the confines of SB8, this model was a success. Chloe told us that the Hotline was able to cover the complete cost of care for everyone in Texas that could be seen by NAF-member clinics, all of whom were complying with SB8. She was rightfully proud of that achievement: "It is a stunning amount of patients that they are able to provide care for, which is wonderful." This number is particularly surprising because NAF expected the overall number of abortions in Texas to decrease by 70 percent because of SB8, but with the Hotline's funding help, and the courageous work of Texas's clinics and abortion supporters, that decrease was only 50 percent.

For patients beyond the SB8 limit, the Hotline helped with travel and other resources. For some patients, this allowed them to get to neighboring states for care. With money and connections to on-the-ground organizations, the Hotline staffers were able to help transport patients to other states and help them navigate those states' barriers, such as waiting periods or other onerous restrictions.

For other patients, however, getting assistance from a national organization like the Hotline was difficult. Rachel told us, "The cases where we most routinely see ourselves running up against a brick wall are cases where, as a national organization, you can throw all the money possible at a situation and it doesn't eviscerate all the boundaries. For example, patients who have chaotic home lives, or are parents with very little support." Rachel continued, "We're a national organization, so I can't walk over to somebody's house and babysit their kid. I can't pick them up and drive them from point A to point B so that they can get to the bus stop. We certainly do our best, and we found some interesting and innovative ways to expand our services like offering food stipends to patients and things like that to try to stop up some of these gaps. But there are just some things where a patient's life, the circumstances that are in their life, it's not conducive to walk away from that for forty-eight to seventy-two hours to go receive care."

Even with all the help they provided, Rachel, Chloe, and their colleagues were keenly aware of the pain and disruption SB8 caused. Before SB8, it was legal for people to get care in their home state with straightforward medical care. Most were able to receive care without crossing state lines, despite the unnecessary barriers they had to overcome because of

Texas restrictions in place long before 2021. But under SB8, even with help from the Hotline, the entire process was drawn out days or even weeks, pushing people later into pregnancy for care and complicating their lives even more because of the logistics and time of travel.

The Texas pre-*Dobbs* experience showed that concentrated hotline assistance could blunt the harm of a law like SB8, but Chloe and Rachel worried about how much this model could be replicated when a dozen or more states ban abortion. They knew that the logistics of coordinating care and funding would become that much more complicated, creating major staffing challenges. Rachel asked rhetorically, for all of the patients who will need help after the decision, the question was "How do we provide individualized flight itineraries and travel plans, let alone just the raw financial resources?"

Two other events before *Dobbs* gave Chloe and Rachel an opportunity to prepare for the onslaught. First, a month and a half before *Dobbs*, Oklahoma enacted a law similar to SB8 allowing for private lawsuits targeting abortion providers and helpers, but starting at conception rather than six weeks of pregnancy, which shut down abortion provision entirely in the state. Oklahoma had been a state where many Texans had been fleeing to obtain an abortion; now, with Oklahoma under the same legal regime, people had to travel even farther.

Second, when the *Dobbs* opinion was leaked, the Hotline was given what Rachel called a "sneak preview" of what to expect almost two months ahead of time. This allowed the Hotline to ramp up its preparations even more. Rachel said that they were able to "expedite and solidify what we needed to do. We were already in the early stages of making some transitions to our patient experience flow to make things simpler, easier, and also reflective of what shifting access would look like. The leak gave us a heads-up and a two-month head start."

In anticipation of the ruling, the Hotline created a better call routing system that more efficiently connected callers with someone who was part of the Hotline's regional case management system. "By doing better call routing," Rachel explained, "we're able to make sure that people are connected with the person who is actually authorized to give them the answer." People working in a particular regional group develop expertise for that area of the country, not only in understanding the law and knowing the clinics in those areas but also in developing relationships with local funds and facilities there. Rachel said, "It's a really big benefit to not have to know everything about all states." Staffing for the regional groups has been fluid because of the frequent changes in state abortion law. But being "nimble," as Rachel put it, has allowed the Hotline to adjust quickly as needs evolve.

When *Dobbs* hit, the Hotline stayed open and was able to meet the surge in callers. The Hotline was able to help everyone with abortion funding for at least a base-level amount of assistance. The amount can go higher, depending on a patient's situation. Hotline staffers do what they can to leverage connections to help with the cost of the abortion in other ways. In the case of Hotline staffers assisting patients who are just a little bit short of funds to pay for the abortion, Rachel said, "You might call the facility that you have a great relationship with, talk to your contact who you speak with two or three times a day, and see if you can make some sort of an arrangement. Maybe a little bit of a clinic discount in exchange for a little bit more funding."

Hotline staffers also try to tap into other resources beyond NAF's own fundraising from donors. Rachel explained: "You might call your contact at a local fund and see if they might be able to contribute. You might talk to the patient and see if they have anything to contribute and if that amount should go toward the cost of the procedure, or if maybe you rec-ommend that they reserve that for some sort of travel-related expense."

Finding funds for travel support post-*Dobbs* was more difficult. Even though the Hotline has increased the amount of travel support it provides, it wasn't able to meet 100 percent of the demand. Such an amount "is so astronomical that it's not even realistic to pitch to donors," Rachel said. The Hotline has begun to develop some relationships with hotels in key locations that have treated patients with dignity, and that connection has helped with some costs. But even with these relationships, the Hotline needs to triage travel funding. It has developed certain policies and con-ditions for travel assistance so that it can help as many people as possible, but it must make many case-by-case decisions about what it can and can-not fund.

Travel support also differs from abortion-funding support in that it is much more labor intensive, involving booking flights, arranging for gas money, helping people with travel glitches of various kinds, and, as Rachel described it, "walking people step-by-step" through the phases of their journey. "We've had conversations with patients at airports where they show up and they brought the wrong bag and it's too big and we're trying to negotiate with them on what to leave and what to bring. Or telling somebody who's never flown before, 'Please don't bring your own shampoo. You're not going to get through security.' TSA is not intuitive, right? We've had instances where we're on the phone with hotels because somebody post-procedure has bled through the sheets and now we're paying a cleanup fee for that."

Supporting so many patients with travel following *Dobbs* taught Chloe and Rachel an important lesson for this new era—that far more than the expected number of patients chose driving over flying, even for very long distances. "We're now seeing people travel unbelievable distances by car," Rachel noted. They prefer driving over flying for many reasons: "Since we exclusively work with a population that falls on the lower end of the socioeconomic spectrum, there's a good chunk of the patient population that work with that has never flown. You also need certain types of identification in order to fly." Beyond these barriers, Rachel highlighted the logistical problems with flight, particularly with what she and others call "the last mile." "Even if we can get you on a flight, how are you getting to the airport? And then, importantly, once you're out of the airport, how are you actually getting to the hotel or to the appointment? So, there's a little bit of a gap that also needs to be solved." Flights also make it more difficult to bring companions, like family or friends, as well as food, water, and other necessities that can make travel less expensive.

With *Dobbs* in place, Chloe and Rachel were able to observe the countrywide ripple effect of abortion bans and the impact that has had on funding and support. "Now it's not just Texas and it's not just Oklahoma," Rachel said while contemplating all of the states that ban abortion post-*Dobbs*. "It's Florida limiting their gestational age down to fifteen weeks. It's Georgia limiting down to six. Georgia was a major hub, so that's been a huge ripple effect." She described other states, such as Kentucky and Wisconsin, that are banning abortion and said, "We're now seeing more and more of these ripples coming out and they're overlapping in a way where access is becoming increasingly stratified, but also really concentrated in just a few major areas."

Chloe and Rachel repeatedly referred to New Mexico, Colorado, Illinois, and North Carolina (before it enacted its twelve-week ban) as being the post-*Dobbs* "stars" that have handled the influx of patients from states with bans. Other states that prepared for a huge influx, such as California and New York, have seen an increase, but the post-*Dobbs* numbers were not as much as some people expected. Travel distance is the reason, Chloe and Rachel explained. Those states are serving an important role post-*Dobbs*, but because they are not as close to states with bans as other states, "they are not what is the difference between access and non-access." Compounding the difficulties is that both California and New York are expensive and large, making travel difficult. "If you're used to more rural areas," Chloe said, "I think you're going to go somewhere that feels more manageable."

Chloe and Rachel explained further that the level of care callers from states with bans need in this new environment impacts other patients the Hotline helps. What they learned from the SB8 experience is that providing the in-depth help needed for patients in states with bans takes time and resources away from patients in other states that the Hotline continues to help. "These patients," Rachel said, referring to people in states with bans, "are now taking the financial energy, resources, staffing time, and logistical coordination that has typically only been reserved for patients who are at the later stages of pregnancy where abortion options start to really become restrictive," Rachel said.

Given the unprecedented legal changes *Dobbs* precipitated, the Hotline was thrust into the spotlight regarding the legality of its operations. Chloe felt she personally was at low risk because she is removed from direct patient interaction. Rachel said that she has thought of her position in the situation in "such a professional context" that she has "bulldozed through the whole thing without giving it too much thought."

But the legal situation is different for an organization such as the Hotline. The precarious issue for the Hotline in the months immediately after *Dobbs* was the legality of funding patients who left their home state to obtain abortion pills and then would return to their home state, where abortion was banned. Chloe and Rachel wouldn't tell us about the organization's internal deliberations and line-drawing, other than being very clear that they have no geographic restrictions on the people with whom they work (whereas they followed restrictions posed by individual state laws on the point in pregnancy after which abortion was illegal).

The guiding principle, Rachel told us, has been "how do we make sure that whatever we do and whatever our approach is, we are remaining viable for as many callers as possible?" And one of the ways they've decided to serve the most people is to follow the law precisely. To Chloe and Rachel, that is how the Hotline remains sustainable, because if it were caught in legal trouble, that would threaten all the help it can provide.

But they did stress that as much as their thinking about legality focused on their continued ability to help the most patients get care, they had to also think about their staff. "It's incredibly important that we protect them and make sure they feel comfortable working here," Chloe said, "so we've been making that the priority." Some of the decisions the Hotline made about how exactly it was going to dispense its funds faced public criticism. "We are all flying by the seat of our pants right now," Rachel said. "We're really trying to do our best during an unprecedented situation. I think that's what I keep going back to, is that people are going to come to slightly different answers on what's the best way to handle it."

Of course, as with everyone, resources were on Chloe's and Rachel's minds each time we talked with them. They know that the funding required to help people from so many states travel much longer distances was virtually immeasurable. Chloe estimated, before *Dobbs*, that the Hotline would need tens of millions of dollars per month to manage the disruption caused by abortion bans. Once *Dobbs* was decided, the deluge of people calling the Hotline was difficult. The Hotline worked on a "first-come, first-served basis," offering as many resources as were needed to callers who reached them in the order they called. But there are limits. "It's an ongoing conversation," Rachel said. "We're really trying to think through what are we going to need to do to really stretch our resources as much as possible."

Navigating this new restrictive environment for the people working the Hotline has been "intense," Rachel said. The calls are longer. The problems people face are more complex. The logistical challenges are sometimes intractable, and the emotional toll is high. "Staff are reporting that just the heaviness of conversations has increased," Rachel said. "There's increased desperation on behalf of callers. The proportion of calls right now of people who are really in crisis and really desperate and don't have a starting point has really increased." But staff members are also thrilled when state laws, internal policies, or funding levels change so that they can offer more assistance. Referring to the week in November 2022 when Georgia's six-week limit was put on hold by a state court, Rachel said, "When we posted internally that we're funding in Georgia up to the pre-*Dobbs* state limits, all we got is heart emojis, excited emojis" in response from the staff.

SUPPORT FOR ABORTION LATER IN PREGNANCY

Abortion later in pregnancy, particularly after viability of the fetus, is very rare—before *Dobbs*, only about 1 percent of abortions in the United States occur after twenty-one weeks' gestation (which is still usually three weeks before viability).[6] But for patients who seek out that care, it has always been difficult to obtain. Part of the reason is that before *Dobbs* there were only four or five abortion clinics that provided care into the third trimester.[7] That number has grown in the past two years, but even with that growth, there are only roughly a dozen clinics in the country where people can get care after twenty-four weeks of pregnancy and fewer still that provide care after twenty-eight weeks.[8] What this means for patients who don't happen to live near one of these clinics is they are going to have to travel, and for some, that travel is going to involve very long distances.

That's where Odile Schalit comes in. When we talked with Odile, she was the executive director of the Brigid Alliance. The national organization, named after a seventh-century saint who, legend has it, helped women who no longer wanted to be pregnant, provides practical support to people who have to travel long distances to access abortion care, especially later in pregnancy.[9] Founded in 2018, Brigid (as it is commonly known) began by assisting patients who were traveling to New York City for care but then quickly branched out to work with clinics across the country that offered care later in pregnancy. The organization leaves abortion funding to other groups but provides customized wraparound service to support patient travel. As Odile explained, "What we're doing is this kind of holistic form of practical support where you get a person who's a coordinator, and they work with you to plan your whole trip and then they're with you at every step of the way supporting you as your situation may change."

As an example of the work Brigid does, Odile told us about one patient she was working with in July 2022, the month after *Dobbs* was decided. "I've been working with someone for the last two weeks who is traveling from Galveston to Boulder, and her appointment is next week. She was referred to us three weeks ago. So three weeks ago I got on the phone with her. I did intake. I planned out her trip. I circled back to her to confirm she liked that, and I've been checking in with her every week since to make sure she knows that we're still here. And today I've been playing phone tag with her to make sure that she has all the information she needs so she's set to travel on Monday. On Monday, I will call her to confirm she's set to travel. On Tuesday, I'll confirm she got to the appointment. And then once we know what day she's done with her appointment, I'll book her return travel, book her local transportation to get there, and make sure she's reimbursed for anything that she needs to be."

Odile came to this intensive work supporting patient travel from her lifelong fascination with reproductive health. In school, she was interested in mental health generally but then began focusing on parent-child relationships, child development, and community health. After a brief stint working in film and television, she went to school for social work and became a doula, a coach for pregnant women. She explained to us that there was a relationship between the two worlds of film and social work: In film, she said, "my entire job was supporting people to feel like their best selves, so that they could perform in the way that they wanted to." As a social worker and doula, Odile saw herself in the same role.

At first Odile was a birth doula. From there she branched out into becoming an abortion doula, working at Planned Parenthood in New York assisting people who had abortions. While in that job, she became passionate about reproductive justice. She saw, in her words, "that having an abortion is an incredible opportunity to bring in the love and care and quality of care that everyone deserves to have throughout their entire lives."

She also saw how people who need an abortion require other forms of support beyond the medical care provided in the clinic. So she came back to the question that she asked herself throughout her professional career: "What are the practical, and emotional, and environmental needs that, when met, support people in feeling whole, feeling safe, and experiencing what autonomy really is in our most beautiful imagination of it?" That life-organizing question for Odile led her to Brigid: she helped launch the organization and a year later became its executive director.

Before *Dobbs*, Brigid was helping ninety to one hundred people per month who had to travel on average around a thousand miles. When the organization began, it partnered with a small group of New York clinics, but it eventually broadened its reach to work with other clinics for patients who need the help. As Odile described it, the only real criterion is, for patients who need later abortion care, whether travel is a barrier. If it is, Brigid will help them, no matter how long-distance the travel is. Odile explained that while local practical support organizations are "vital and unique" in helping with local or even medium-distance travel, "Brigid focuses its services and skills on longer-distance travel. Of those organizations that can do this type of expensive and complex travel support, there are very few."

Anticipating an influx of need because of *Dobbs* looming, in the beginning of 2022, Brigid started preparing for expansion. They worked on building out their technology, training new staff, bolstering security, memorializing their training into an easily-accessible manual, and creating protocols so that staff don't have to reinvent the wheel with each caller.

This preparation proved essential in handling the post-*Dobbs* crunch. By the time we talked with Odile for the third time, in January 2023, Brigid's monthly volume had doubled since right before *Dobbs*. The organization was now helping almost two hundred people per month. Part of that increase was due to states banning abortion, creating a greater need for long-distance travel. Part was due to an increase in the number of people needing later abortion care due to delays associated with bans. And part of that was due to a decrease in the number of providers offering later third-trimester care. "It's still an intense time," Odile told us. "We have most definitely not felt as a community that the patterns of patient access have settled. They're still evolving."

Odile offered an example to explain the impact of *Dobbs* on Brigid's work. Before *Dobbs*, even though abortion was highly regulated in a state like Alabama, clinics in those states provided care up to twenty weeks of pregnancy. Now, post-*Dobbs*, a patient in the state who needs care in the weeks leading up to the twentieth week can't get care in their home state. "'I'm twenty weeks pregnant, I live in Alabama, and I can't get an abortion. Where am I going to go?'" Odile said, referring to a typical case. Now, she continued, there are so many more steps for the patient to navigate. "Figuring out where a clinic is. Figuring out funding. Figuring out who provides funding, getting that funding, figuring out who provides practical support, getting that practical support. All for an appointment that may be several weeks out because all these clinics are getting backed up." For people in these situations, Odile summarized, "the pathway is intensified."

The work to plan and coordinate this kind of long-distance travel is labor intensive. This travel is usually by air, so Brigid staffers work with the patient and the clinic to facilitate transportation to and from the airport, flights, overnight stays, food, childcare, and anything else the patient needs to make the travel possible. Each time we talked with Odile, she stressed that Brigid had the money to support all the patients referred to the organization but didn't "have enough time in the day" to do so. "It's not about money, it's not about desire. It's literally about not enough time in the day, not enough hands in the pot to get it done and to do it well." She continued, "We only have so many people and there are now so many folks who need our services."

SB8 gave Brigid, like the other organizations discussed in this chapter, a head start in thinking about the issues *Dobbs* was going to present. In particular, Brigid used the opportunity to think deeply about legal risk, particularly as an organization with staff in many different states, including states with bans. Because of SB8, the organization worked with a law firm, paid for by a donor, to determine the best way to safely help Texans travel out of state for care. That review expanded to a fifty-state review in anticipation of *Dobbs*.

The week after *Dobbs* was, as Odile described it, "a shit show." The organization had watched one of the essential Texas funds close its doors right before *Dobbs*. That "had a ripple effect across abortion funds and practical support organizations." Brigid did not want to follow suit, but it became apparent that the organization's legal analysis of its own post–*Dobbs* risk was not going to be finished before *Dobbs* was decided. Odile lamented, "We made the really hard choice to shut down for a week, which sucked, but also felt really important that we just make sure we feel really clear about how we're moving forward."

Knowing that the organization was going to shut down temporarily, Brigid supported as many people as possible with high-dollar grants in the weeks right before *Dobbs*: "We were pre-booking travel and pre-paying for hotels," Odile told us, "because the fear was that if we close, and the analysis is that if we've paid for any services post-*Dobbs* that we're violating a law, then that's a problem. So we were trying to get our money out to our clients and pay for things before that date."

Even though everyone at the organization knew ahead of time of the decision to close, implementing it was difficult and emotional. Odile found it hard to describe that moment to us even a month later. She choked up when she said, about the day *Dobbs* was decided, "Friday came and it happened. The staff knew that they needed to log out of the database, log out of their email, and then meet up in a group meeting an hour later." Everyone was, as Odile recalled, "devastated." Staff who helped clients were no longer able to do so, while staff who talked to press and donors became overwhelmed with the attention the organization attracted in the wake of *Dobbs*. Everyone would have preferred to be able to continue to help clients, especially in this moment.

When the organization reopened a week after the decision, the national landscape was "absolute mayhem," said Odile. The staff leapt into action. Partner clinics referred patients to Brigid who had needed assistance during the week. Odile said that she thought "we were still able to help the majority of the people that were referred to us because it was only one week." In retrospect, she thinks the "impact of our closure was really pretty insignificant," but it was demoralizing to be unable to help patients during such an intense time.

The staff reaction to the pause was mixed: "They hated that we would have to do this for their clients," Odile said, "but I think they felt protected and cared for and grateful." After the week's pause, Odile was very proud that Brigid resumed assisting patients from all fifty states.

Even with all this work being done by Brigid and similar organizations, Odile is concerned about the women who inevitably are going to fall through the cracks. "I am concerned with people who are isolated due to physical or developmental impairments. I'm worried about people who are undocumented, who are in violent relationships, who live in rural areas." People can only get help if they know, or are told about, organizations that can help them. Despite the resources and commitment of the people profiled in this chapter and those like them, some people just won't be able to get the support they need.

SUSTAINABILITY

According to data from the Guttmacher Institute, in the first half of 2023, roughly double the number of women traveled across state lines to get an abortion as before *Dobbs*.[10] Nearly 1 in 5 people who obtained an abortion in the formal healthcare sector in the first half of 2023, about 92,000 people, crossed state lines compared to 1 in 10, or about 41,000, before *Dobbs*. At the same time, if 1 in 5 abortion patients travel from out of state for an abortion, that means 4 out of 5 patients don't. In other words, it is clear—given that the number of abortions overall has increased in the aftermath of *Dobbs*—that both interstate travelers *and* women who reside in states where abortion remains legal are being supported in this new environment.

The influx of money pouring into abortion funds and practical support organizations as a result of *Dobbs* has helped all patients, not just interstate travelers. The only reason this money has had an impact in supporting high numbers of people traveling both long-distance and locally seeking abortion care is because of the work of Oriaku, Chloe, Rachel, Odile, and the many people like them around the country who support abortion patients in this new restrictive environment.

All these people were proud of this post-*Dobbs* patient support work. Given the reported numbers showing a slight increase in abortions in the months right after the Supreme Court decision, they were justified in feeling that way. Yet, each of the people we talked with expressed significant concerns about sustainability. "The explosion in need is so severe," Rachel told us. "Currently, demand is exceeding our resources, so we're just trying to do the best we can."

When we talked with Oriaku at the end of 2022, they told us that the spike in donations and attention post-*Dobbs* helped NNAF meet its 2022 fundraising goals by September. But Oriaku stressed to us and to everyone they talk with that "this is an anomaly. We cannot make the assumption that funding is going to consistently be like this. We want it to happen, but that's work that we have to do to get it there." Oriaku hopes that *Dobbs* and the surrounding attention on abortion is a "wake-up call for more investment" in patient support, funding, and access. But while they wait to see if that happens, NNAF's budget for 2023 did not increase, despite the increased donations in 2022, because of the lack of certainty about what donations would look like a year or more after *Dobbs*.

Like NNAF, Brigid also experienced an overwhelming surge in financial support because of *Dobbs*. Nonetheless, Odile was not sure about the future. "I mean, honestly, I'm pretty concerned it's not going to be sustained," she said. Speaking for almost everyone doing the intensive work of supporting patients post-*Dobbs*, Odile said, "There's still this tension and fear that people are going to stop watching."

CHAPTER EIGHT

ABORTION'S UNCERTAIN FUTURE

We're doing this no matter what.

—ORIAKU NJOKU, National Network
of Abortion Funds

A new chapter in the story of abortion in America is upon us. *Dobbs* overturned *Roe v. Wade*, ending a constitutional right to abortion for now, but so far, because of everything we chronicle in this book, abortion has continued to be available for most people. Indeed, much to the surprise of many—including the two of us—the best data we have so far reveals that the number of abortions performed in the United States has *increased* after the decision.[1]

The stories profiled in this book explain this seemingly counterintuitive development. *Dobbs* was supposed to dramatically decrease the number of abortions in America, but the hard, nimble, and creative work of the providers where clinics have remained open, the growth and new delivery models of abortion pills, and the never-ending work of those advocates who help with abortion travel and funding refused to let that happen. This continuity of care is cause for celebration in the face of a devastating blow from the Supreme Court.

The people profiled in this book, and others like them on the ground throughout the country, are staring adversity in the eye and telling it not now, not for the people we serve. Their resolve is exceeded only by the determination of pregnant people in states where abortion is banned to nonetheless get the care they need and find a way to have an abortion, either by traveling to a legal state or obtaining abortion pills through various channels.

The truth is that this has long been the story of abortion in this country and throughout the world. Even before *Roe v. Wade*, when abortion was illegal in the United States, women still obtained abortions and doctors and others still provided them. There was legal and reputational risk for the people providing abortions, and sometimes, there was safety risk for the people obtaining them in less-than-ideal situations. When *Roe* made abortion legal throughout the United States, these particular risks largely disappeared, but because of the increasing unnecessary regulations and restrictions affecting abortion in some states, women still had to push through many obstacles to get an abortion. And they did.

We have seen the same around the world. In countries where abortion is illegal, women still get abortions, through abortion pills and other means. Despite tens of thousands of women dying from illegal abortion worldwide each year, the basic human need to control reproduction has proved time and time again that abortion can't and won't be stopped.[2]

The story since the Supreme Court overturned *Roe* in 2022 has been much the same. The risks are different, and the exact abortion service delivery mechanisms vary, but the overall point is one that we should have seen coming, even if we didn't: the resilience of those seeking and providing abortion is unflagging. Combine that resilience with a profound resistance to removing a nationally recognized fundamental right, and we have an explanation of what we are seeing now in the increase in abortion numbers despite the Supreme Court's decision. Everyone featured in this book fills in the details of the story that the numbers tell.

But as much as this is an unexpected and exciting development in the face of a ground-shifting Supreme Court decision, the celebration must be muted, for several reasons. First and foremost, even though abortion has remained more available than originally feared, *Dobbs* has brought changes and disruptions to people's lives and well-being that are unacceptable. Abortion patients should not have to take cross-country flights or drive hundreds of miles and lose much-needed wages to get healthcare—care that in a rational society would be affordable and available in their own communities. Doctors and other clinicians who have the skills and experience to care for patients should not have to face the wrenching decision to leave communities to which they are deeply attached. Clinic staff in surge states should not have to work punishing hours to accommodate floods of desperate out-of-towners. And abortion funders and practical support groups should not have to spend valuable resources helping people get care that should be delivered close to home and with government support. As a bottom-line nonnegotiable principle, women and other pregnancy-capable people, no matter where they live, should not be prevented from being fully participating citizens in the public sphere—something that is only possible with control of one's reproduction.

Thinking more broadly, there are important parts of the story that go beyond what is covered in this book. Inevitably, despite the efforts of everyone in this book and those like them, there will be people left out who are unable to obtain an abortion. For those people, the consequences can be severe. Also, in this post-*Dobbs* landscape, women facing emergency pregnancy conditions are suffering in ways that are made even more difficult because of the lack of a national right to abortion. In addition, the removal of this national right increases the risk that people seeking abortion will be caught up in the criminal justice system, especially those who are, statistically, its most common target—people of color and low-income people.

There are consequences for the healthcare system as well. The increase in medication abortion, especially outside the traditional healthcare system, complicates the narrative that abortion is healthcare, a conviction that has been at the heart of abortion rights and justice advocacy for decades. Abortion bans also are having a negative impact on the availability of non-abortion obstetric and gynecological care, resulting in doctors and other healthcare professionals fleeing states with bans.

And everything we have written about throughout this book and in this conclusion is subject to an uncertain future. The 2024 election along with ongoing legal battles could drastically change the underlying landscape. So could a drop in funding and other resources for all of the types of support discussed in this book. Since *Dobbs*, support has been flowing to organizations doing the work, but if that tapers off, as data collected in the first half of 2024 seem to indicate, the future could look very different. In the remainder of this chapter we discuss these unfolding consequences as part of the widespread fallout from *Dobbs* and speculate about the future of abortion going forward.

THOSE LEFT OUT

Post-*Dobbs*, abortion numbers are up. Many people who now live in states with an abortion ban face serious disruption to their lives to get an abortion—travel, time off work, finding someone to accompany them, navigating unfamiliar locations, contacting multiple different support organizations, spending money on food and lodging. These disruptions are greater than the obstacles they faced before *Dobbs*, but many are still finding a way.

But not everyone. Even though abortion numbers have increased over-all, no study has found that everyone who would have sought and obtained an abortion before *Dobbs* has been able to do so since then. In fact, anecdotal evidence points to a substantial number of people who have been unable to obtain an abortion and have had to carry their pregnancies to term. Initial studies in this uncertain environment support this inference. For instance, a study released in late 2023 found that there was a 2.3 percent increase in births in states with abortion bans post-*Dobbs*, resulting in an additional thirty thousand babies born per year.[3] That this number isn't higher is the big post-*Dobbs* surprise, but it is still a significant number, meaning many people have been left behind because of the barriers to care that exist because of *Dobbs*.

The Supreme Court's unjust ruling has forced these individuals to remain pregnant and give birth against their will, leading to increased risk of poor life consequences. Maternal mortality rates, already shocking in the United States when compared to those of other industrialized nations, have been predicted by scholars to rise as a consequence of *Dobbs*. Though precise data on this question are not yet available, one study predicts that maternal mortality could rise by 24 percent because of the decision.[4] This anticipated rise is especially germane for Black women who already have maternal mortality rates four times those of white women.[5]

But beyond the risk of death, the landmark Turnaway Study has shown the significant costs involved in being denied a desired abortion. As we discussed in the introduction, the study found that, compared to those who received an abortion, women who were unable to access one were more likely to stay mired in poverty, remain tethered to an abusive part-ner, have worse physical health, have lower career and life aspirations, and experience worse maternal bonding with their children, among other consequences.[6] That fewer people than expected fall into this group is great news post-*Dobbs*, but there are still some who do, and for those people these consequences will be life-changing.

It should come as no surprise who is most likely to fall into this group. Consistent with the long history of race-based inequities in this country, more than half of Black women of reproductive age in this country live in states where abortion is banned, likely to be banned, or heavily restricted.[7]

But the impact of abortion bans is much broader. The group of people who are most unable to get an abortion after *Dobbs* includes the most vulnerable women in society: those in severe poverty, who may not have a computer or any other means to even know where they could get help finding and financing an abortion; those who don't have the resources necessary for multiday travel, such as a working car, long-distance gas money, and money to eat away from home for multiple meals; those for whom losing even one or two days of work runs the risk of job loss; those without the family or financial resources to arrange childcare for their children if they have to leave their state, especially if their abortion involves an overnight stay; racial and religious minorities who feel unsafe traveling into parts of the country with which they lack familiarity and where they fear increased racism and bias; undocumented people for whom plane travel is impossible and for whom even long car trips can be risky; those living in domestic abuse situations, whose partners have taken away their identification documents or track their every move; those with disabilities who have long faced challenges accessing care in stand-alone clinics; minors who still, in many locations, are forced by law to involve their parents in their decision; and those who are incarcerated, who face challenges accessing quality medical care of all kinds, including abortion care.

Now that the Supreme Court has overruled *Roe*, these are the individuals who are most likely to suffer the consequences the Turnaway Study warned about. Which means these are the people who are bearing most of the brunt of *Dobbs*, even if for so many other people abortion remains attainable.

EMERGENCY ABORTIONS

Almost immediately after *Dobbs*, stories began to proliferate through media outlets of wanted pregnancies gone wrong and women being denied emergency medical care because of abortion bans. These stories have continued to dominate the news around abortion post-*Dobbs*.

For instance, Kate Cox made national headlines in late 2023 when she sued the state of Texas to get an abortion.[8] At twenty weeks Kate's fetus was diagnosed with a fatal fetal anomaly. Kate wanted an abortion, not just because the condition was incompatible with life but also because her medical history made carrying the pregnancy to term risky. Having already had two cesarean section births, Kate was at risk of uterine rupture if she carried to term, and she was also experiencing other serious pregnancy complications.

So Kate did something that almost no other adult women have done in the past half century—while pregnant, she filed a lawsuit seeking a court order giving her the right to get an abortion. In Texas, the abortion ban has an exception for a "life-threatening condition," and Kate's lawyers argued that her situation qualified. She was immediately successful before the trial court, but the Texas attorney general appealed while threatening legal action against any hospital and doctor who performed an abortion for Kate in the meantime. While waiting for the Texas Supreme Court to rule, Kate and her lawyers made the difficult decision to travel out of state to get an abortion rather than wait for the state high court to rule and risk further health consequences. When it did rule, the Texas Supreme Court found that Kate had not met the requirements for the state's abortion ban exception. The court wrote that "some difficulties in pregnancy, however, even serious ones, do not pose the heightened risks to the mother that the exception encompassed."[9]

Such stories—like that of Amanda Zurawski, discussed in the introduction, who developed sepsis from an emergency complication during her wanted pregnancy—have resonated with the American public in a deep way and have driven much of the discourse post-*Dobbs*. Individuals across all social class lines and income levels whose pregnancies have gone horribly wrong have experienced enormous difficulties because of *Dobbs*. In this book we have focused primarily on nonemergency abortions that take place either in clinics or at home with pills obtained online—that is, "ordinary" abortions available to largely healthy people who do not want to be pregnant. People with serious medical complications from pregnancy who need an abortion constitute a minority of abortion patients.

But for this small group of pregnant people who are experiencing medical emergencies, an in-hospital abortion is typically necessary to preserve their health and even their lives. And for such patients who live in states that have banned abortion, the situation since *Dobbs* has in many instances been a nightmare.

Prior to *Dobbs*, those facing some of the most serious problems of pregnancy—such as ectopic pregnancies (where a fertilized egg implants outside the uterus) or PPROM (pre-term pre-labor rupture of membranes, known colloquially as a pregnant woman's "water breaking," which can lead to a septic infection) and others—would typically receive abortions, even in states hostile to abortion, as such conditions are known to be life-threatening. Such abortions in conservative regions often were referred to as "terminations," and the doctors who performed the procedures did not necessarily identify as "abortion providers."

States banning abortion in the wake of *Dobbs* have made it impossible to continue this previous arrangement of quietly taking care of such emergencies. The situation since the decision can be described only as legal chaos, with doctors and other hospital personnel confused and at odds as to what is permissible. Theoretically, each of the states with an abortion ban permits an abortion when the patient's life is threatened, but what this exception actually means in practice is a highly subjective matter. As Lisa Harris, an obstetrician-gynecologist at the University of Michigan and a national thought leader in abortion care wrote in anticipation of *Dobbs*, "What does the risk of death have to be, and how imminent must it be? Might abortion be permissible in a patient with pulmonary hypertension, for whom we cite a 30-to-50% chance of dying with ongoing pregnancy? Or must it be 100%?"[10]

An answer to this question has never been legally clarified, and the statutory exception language varies dramatically from state to state.[11] Often it is hospital counsel, not healthcare professionals, who makes the final decision as to whether an abortion may proceed under a state's law. Researchers at the University of California, San Francisco, have investigated how treatment of those with problem pregnancies has changed as a result of *Dobbs*. The Care Post-Roe study has documented that clinicians treating such patients experience anguish at the shocking risks to which their patients were subjected, as different parties within the hospital setting could not agree on whether to allow abortions that had once been the standard of care within the field of obstetrics.[12] Clinicians reported, for instance, having to delay or deny care because fetal cardiac activity was still present, despite patients facing serious health risks that can lead to death or serious health consequences. The study also collected testimonies from clinicians about women denied abortion who were carrying fetuses already in demise or with conditions that made it likely that if the pregnancy were to result in a birth, the newborn would shortly suffer a painful death.

As doctors, lawyers, and administrators quarrel over what treatment is permitted and when it can be offered, these situations inevitably have led to previously unimaginable scenarios for patients. For instance, in Oklahoma a woman had a partial molar pregnancy—an abnormal form of pregnancy in which a nonviable fertilized egg implants in the uterus; pregnancies with this condition do not result in a healthy baby and could put the woman's life at risk. As reported by *The Guardian*, she was told by hospital officials that "they could not provide an abortion until she was actively crashing in front of them or on the verge of a heart attack. In the meantime, the best that they could offer was to let [her] sit in the parking lot so that she would be close to the hospital when her condition further deteriorated."[13]

In early 2024, the *New Yorker* reported on the first documented case of a death of a young woman resulting from a state abortion ban. Though there is no indication in the Texas woman's medical records that she requested an abortion, medical experts interviewed for the story agreed that terminating her pregnancy was clearly indicated based on her dangerously high blood pressure during the pregnancy; however, because of the state's abortion ban, no one discussed it with her.[14] While this abortion-related tragedy was among the very first post-*Dobbs* deaths to be documented, some observers speculate that more such deaths have occurred but have not been publicized.

An obvious reason that there has been such hesitation to treat such serious cases is the stiff penalties state legislatures have imposed on those who perform abortions that are not permitted by the law. In the most extreme cases, Texas and Alabama permit prison sentences of up to life imprisonment, heavy fines, and loss of medical licenses for those who violate the states' laws. Sympathetic doctors in these states who do not want to risk crossing the line and possibly losing their livelihood and their freedom have coped with this situation in the best way they can, given their limited options. They have established informal networks of communication with colleagues in states where abortion remains legal and have arranged for patients in crisis to travel there, often by ambulance if necessary. This out-of-state travel for those in physical, and often emotional, crisis is obviously not the way healthcare should operate in a civilized society, especially where resources and expertise are available to treat these women in their own communities.

As a result of these terrible stories, one of the unintended consequences of *Dobbs* has been that it has brought to the fore what had previously been less visible to the general public: although most pregnancies proceed uneventfully, a not-insignificant minority of pregnancies can be extremely dangerous. It has been known throughout history that childbirth can be dangerous to a woman's life, and despite huge advances in obstetrics, child-birth is still fourteen times as likely to lead to death as abortion.[15] This fact of life, and death, led Warren Hern, a longtime abortion doctor in the United States, to write: "Pregnancy is dangerous; abortion can be lifesaving."[16] Or, as the sociologist Jocelyn Viterna, in commenting on the callousness shown by the state of Texas toward those experiencing pregnancy-related emer-gencies, pointed out: "Pregnancy remains the most dangerous and com-plicated biological process that humans undertake."[17] Thus, even though emergency pregnancy complications requiring an abortion occur in only a minority of pregnancies, they can occur in any pregnancy. Post-*Dobbs*, the American public is getting a crash course in these realities.

ABORTION *IS* HEALTHCARE

For years, "abortion is healthcare" has been the mantra of abortion sup-porters. This slogan had its origins in the period before and immediately after *Roe*: before the decision, pro-choice forces, in response to the death and injuries of the criminalization era, demanded legalization and incor-poration of abortion care into mainstream medicine; after *Roe* this de-mand continued when it became clear how slowly and ambivalently this normalization was occurring.[18] The arrival of medication abortion in the United States in 2000, particularly the more recent increase in the use of those pills in response to *Dobbs*, has complicated the actual meaning of this demand because an increasing number of people are obtaining abortion pills with very little or no medical professional involvement at all. In short, at first glance the proliferation of medication abortion arguably weakens the demand that abortion be part of the formal healthcare system.

But the aftermath of *Dobbs*, which has seen widespread media cov-erage of the shockingly inadequate treatment of pregnant people need-ing in-hospital treatment, gives a new urgency to the old argument that abortion care is an essential component of modern healthcare. The efforts discussed in chapter 6 to distribute abortion pills in various ways do not undermine the case that abortion is a legitimate part of healthcare; rather, these activities expand the meaning of the saying.

While it is true that more people are managing their abortions outside the traditional healthcare system with the use of abortion pills, many are doing so with the assistance of medical professionals. For instance, the groups offering abortion via telehealth that we have described involve some form of consultation with medical professionals. Furthermore, even women who initially access pills without consulting a medical professional, such as through an online pharmacy or a local informal network, have the option of consulting medical professionals through the Miscarriage and Abortion Hotline and other similar groups if they have any questions or concerns during the process.

Additionally, for the small portion of patients operating completely without assistance of medical professionals who will seek follow-up care to confirm the abortion is complete or because they believe they are experiencing complications, such care will likely involve a medical facility, whether a local doctor's office or an emergency room. Thus, the range of options available to contemporary abortion patients, even with the challenges imposed by *Dobbs*, is consistent with the broader contemporary American healthcare system, where patients often can choose their level of direct contact with medical institutions.

Consider, for instance, a person deciding how to handle an increasingly painful infected cut: that person can use ointment already in the medicine cabinet at home, go to the pharmacy and buy treatments available on the shelf, talk with a medical professional via phone or video call and follow that advice, make an appointment with a local doctor to get care at the office or a prescription, or seek care at a local urgent-care facility or emergency room. In many ways, the options for abortion patients now mirror the options for people seeking care for other health problems.

THE RISK OF CRIMINALIZATION

Of course, the difference between someone managing an infection on their own but eventually going to see a clinician if it gets worse and someone who uses abortion pills outside the formal healthcare system but then seeks medical help if there is too much bleeding is that the latter faces legal risk. The stories of Lizelle Herrera and Brittany Watts demonstrate how patients who have shown up in emergency rooms after using abortion pills or in the midst of a miscarriage—the two situations are, medically, virtually indistinguishable—have been reported to police. Just before *Dobbs* in spring 2022 when Texas's SB8 was in effect but its full abortion ban was not, Lizelle Herrera went to a Texas emergency room because of complications after using abortion pills.[19] A nurse reported her to local authorities who then charged her with murder. The charges were dropped two days later, but her arrest sent shockwaves through a nervous public awaiting the Supreme Court's decision.

In 2023, the stunning case of Brittany Watts highlighted the post-*Dobbs* risk for women undergoing miscarriages.[20] At twenty-two weeks pregnant, experiencing severe abdominal pain, she repeatedly visited a local Catholic hospital, where a doctor found her fetus to be nonviable and urged that labor be induced. While the facility took its time debating the legality of such a move, Watts miscarried at home while sitting on her toilet. She then flushed some of the products of conception and removed others to an outdoor area. Afterwards, she returned to the hospital for post-miscarriage care, but upon telling a nurse of the details of her pregnancy loss, the nurse alerted the police. In what can only be described as a surreal event, the police impounded her toilet, destroying it in the process as they searched for fetal remains. The local prosecutor charged her with "abuse of a corpse," but ultimately the grand jury declined to bring an indictment. Watts's story is why it comes as no surprise that the Care Post-Roe study received several accounts of patients who had flown from states which had banned abortion to legal states for miscarriage care because they were fearful of being accused of attempting an abortion.[21]

To be sure, the problem of the criminalization of pregnancy outcomes is one that predates *Dobbs*. The legal advocacy group Pregnancy Justice found that between 2006 and 2022 there had been 1,400 cases involving pregnancy-related criminalization in the United States (most involving drug use), with poor women and women of color most impacted (as in the cases just described).[22] The post-*Dobbs* era has the potential to greatly exacerbate this problem of criminalization, especially if emergency room staff continue to seek out the criminal justice system rather than focusing on caring for their patients.[23]

TURMOIL IN OBSTETRICS AND GYNECOLOGY

Dobbs's ripple effects have reached well beyond abortion care. The lack of routine abortion training in states with abortion bans (discussed in chapter 2) coupled with the legal and medical uncertainty about the treatment of very ill patients or those carrying severely compromised fetuses has led to worrisome developments within the field of obstetrics and gynecology. There have been repeated reports since *Dobbs* of doctors in the field fleeing states with abortion bans, or planning to do so, because of well-grounded fears that they will be unable to properly take care of their pregnant patients or will be subject to legal sanctions if they do. Many are also concerned that they will not be able to get proper care for their own

or their family members' pregnancies if ever needed. Those who stay report distress over the inability to provide patients the care they need, fear
about the legal risks, and negative mental health effects.[24]

Idaho provides a particularly vivid example of this fallout. Idaho has
a complete abortion ban, which the state supreme court upheld in 2023.[25]
The same year, the state's legislature further cemented its hostility to reproductive health by shutting down its maternal mortality review committee—so far the only state to do so, and this despite the fact that Idaho's
maternal mortality rate is very high.[26] In this hostile environment, within
one year after *Dobbs* five out of the nine maternal fetal medical special-
ists in the state, those who care for women with high-risk pregnancies,
announced that they were leaving the state.[27] Additionally, a number of
obstetrics and gynecology generalists in rural areas of the state have also
left, leading to the closing of a number of maternity-care units in local
hospitals, exacerbating the already existing problem of "obstetrical deserts." These are more prevalent in rural areas and in states that are hostile
to abortion, such as Idaho, where thirteen of the state's forty-four counties
lacked maternity care as of late 2023.[28]

Research has shown, unsurprisingly, that when pregnant people in rural areas do not have ready access to hospitals with maternity units the
outcomes for them and their newborns are worse than in urban popula-
tions.[29] Rural areas also tend to be poorer than urban areas, which adds
layers of hardship. One report on the closure of a maternity service in a
rural county in Idaho told of pregnant patients worried about finding a
car and paying for gas to get to the nearest labor and delivery unit roughly
forty-five miles away. The report also told of a patient who was due to deliver in January, a time of heavy snowfall in the state; the patient planned
to pack supplies such as rubber gloves and a shower curtain in case she had
to deliver on the way to the hospital.[30]

Importantly, in Idaho, none of the physicians fleeing the state identified as "abortion providers." Rather, one can assume, these physicians
realized that the simple fact of being an obstetrician-gynecologist implies
that inevitably some portion of the patient population will need an abortion or care that might tread the line of the state's abortion laws.

Another disturbing sign of the fallout from *Dobbs* is the drop in residency applications to obstetrics and gynecology programs. According to
the American Medical Association, in the 2022–23 residency application

cycle, in states in which abortion had been totally banned, the number of applicants to such programs from medical schools in the United States fell by more than 10 percent in one year.[31] Overall, residency applications to this specialty fell by 5 percent.

In another ominous development, when third- and fourth-year medical students were surveyed in spring 2023, 58 percent of all of the students—not just those planning to go into obstetrics and gynecology—said they were "unlikely or very unlikely" to apply for a residency in a state that had banned abortion.[32] Putting together these related issues of suspended abortion training, doctor flight, and reduced residency applications, the grim future we can foresee for those needing reproductive healthcare in states with abortion bans is fewer doctors in this field, and for those remaining, less knowledge of and experience with the procedures some of their patients will undoubtedly require.

AN UNCERTAIN LEGAL AND POLITICAL FUTURE

The tremendous efforts to keep abortion available for patients that we have detailed in this book are an inspirational counterbalance to the Supreme Court's overturning the fundamental right to abortion that had existed for half a century. As we finished writing this chapter in the middle of 2024, much remained uncertain about the future of abortion in America. It is very possible that court cases and elections on the horizon could change the environment significantly, forcing abortion providers, supporters, advocates, and patients to turn on a dime once again.

On the legal front, even though the Supreme Court justices in the majority in *Dobbs* wrote as if overturning *Roe* would mean that the Court no longer was in the business of officiating legal disputes about abortion, in 2024, the Court once again faced big questions about abortion. In one case, the Court was faced with the question of whether the federal law that requires hospital emergency rooms to treat people presenting with emergency conditions—the Emergency Medical Treatment and Labor Act, or EMTALA—requires emergency rooms to provide an abortion to a patient who is pregnant and suffering serious complications. Texas and Idaho, two states with near-complete abortion bans, separately claimed in federal court that EMTALA never requires an abortion so they can implement their state abortion bans despite the federal law. In June 2024, the Supreme Court surprised everyone and ruled that it had improperly taken Idaho's case, leaving the issue undecided for now. However, sometime in the near future the Court will almost certainly address the issue head-on, as the cases from both states are still working their way through the system.[33]

The issue of emergency abortions that would be required by EMTALA but not allowed under state law exceptions for life-threatening conditions is important, but fortunately the number of people experiencing these types of severe pregnancy emergencies is low. The other case the Supreme Court considered in 2024 had the potential to impact a much larger number of people. In this case a group of antiabortion doctors sought to ban or seriously restrict the use of mifepristone, the first drug in the two-drug regimen for medication abortion. They challenged the FDA's approval of the drug as not based on science. Even though decades of research have shown the drug to be safe and effective, two conservative lower federal courts had agreed with the challengers.

In June 2024, the Supreme Court rejected this challenge, finding that the doctors who brought the case did not have legal standing to do so because they hadn't been personally injured.[34] For now, the case is no longer an immediate threat to medication abortion, but the antiabortion movement has already tried to revive the case with three states as plaintiffs, so the ultimate fate of this strategy is yet unknown as of June 2024.

This strategy of attacking the FDA's approval of mifepristone could have broad impact on abortion accessibility if the courts or the FDA rolls back the clock to a time before the FDA approved mifepristone for remote care. If mifepristone can no longer be dispensed through telehealth, it is possible that abortion providers in the United States would stop providing telehealth abortions. This would have serious consequences for patients' ability to access medication abortion. A recent study found that if telehealth abortion were not available, patients' travel time would be considerably increased, making it more difficult to get a timely abortion. Some people would simply not be able to manage to get an abortion at all. In particular, the study found the elimination of telehealth dispensation of abortion pills would fall hardest on rural patients, those experiencing food insecurity, and younger patients.[35]

Increasing the uncertainty surrounding medication abortion is the possibility that if mifepristone becomes unavailable or further restricted, American abortion providers will switch to a one-drug protocol for medication abortion. Abortion providers around the world use misoprostol alone to induce abortion, as do many people using pills on their own to complete an abortion. The use of misoprostol alone is highly safe and effective and endorsed by leading medical organizations, such as the World Health Organization and the American College of Obstetricians and Gynecologists.[36] Early studies showed that misoprostol alone was somewhat less effective than when used with mifepristone, but more recent studies show that it might be just as effective. However, even if it is as effective when used alone, some side effects might be more pronounced, such as nausea, diarrhea, and cramping, and the process can take longer and need additional doses of the medication.

No matter the outcome of legal challenges or administrative changes to mifepristone, the use of misoprostol by itself would not be affected, as this drug, approved and widely used for ulcer treatments, has not been challenged or questioned. If American providers were to switch to this protocol, telehealth provision of abortion would continue in this country, though it could be viewed as a less desirable option.

These are just a few of the many legal battles around abortion that have played out in the courts post-*Dobbs*. Other cases working their way through state and federal courts are challenging abortion bans and restrictions on state constitutional grounds, arguing that federal approval of mifepristone preempts state bans or restrictions on abortion pills, contesting state limits on interstate travel related to abortion, and more. As all these court battles are waged, the legal playing field upon which all the people in this book operate could be constantly shifting in the coming years.

The political arena features similar uncertainty. Since *Dobbs* was decided in June 2022, American voters have been crystal clear about their outrage that *Roe* was overturned. In August of that year, voters in deeply conservative Kansas overwhelmingly rejected a ballot initiative that would have eliminated abortion rights under the state constitution. Many forecasters expected the antiabortion side to prevail and polls leading up to the vote were close; however, on election day, the abortion rights side won by double digits.

As of spring 2024, there have been six other statewide ballot initiatives focusing on abortion, and the abortion rights position has won each time. These victories have occurred in the conservative states of Kansas, Montana, and Kentucky, in the somewhat purple states of Ohio and Michigan, and the more liberal states of Vermont and California. This unbroken string of success for abortion at the ballot box will be tested in November 2024, when ten states will have abortion initiatives on the ballot.

Voter outrage over *Dobbs* is also widely considered to have been a major factor in Democrats' exceeding expectations and bucking historical trends in the 2022 midterm elections. And in March 2024, in one of the most surprising electoral victories since *Dobbs*, a Democratic candidate in a state legislative district in Alabama that had previously been held by a Republican won in a landslide after campaigning on abortion rights and support for in vitro fertilization. An ad where she told her own abortion story was a central element of her campaign.[37]

The huge questions, of course, are what role abortion will play in the 2024 election and what the outcome of that election will be. Though the electorate has shown itself to be unquestionably in support of legal abortion, especially when it is presented to the voters directly in the form of a single-issue ballot question, it is not clear how that will translate to a presidential election. As of summer 2024, it appears that Democrats are doing everything to foreground issues related to abortion and reproductive rights, hoping that voters will remember that Donald Trump, the Republican nominee, proudly appointed three of the five justices who overturned *Roe* and that Vice President Kamala Harris, the Democratic nominee, has long been a forceful advocate for abortion rights.

At the same time, candidate Trump appears to be doing everything in his power to downplay his role in *Dobbs* and position himself as seeking a middle ground on abortion. If abortion is a decisive issue in the election once again in 2024, Harris and her strongly pro-choice running mate, Tim Walz, should win, and Trump and his virulently antiabortion running mate, J. D. Vance, should lose. But we, of course, have no crystal ball that will tell us the outcome (though by the time you read this, you will know what happened).

A Republican victory for the presidency, especially if it is matched by victories in both the House and Senate, could be disastrous for abortion care in the United States. Republicans have made no secret of their desire to impose further bans on abortion, with some proposing a national ban after the first trimester, others proposing a total ban. Even with complete Republican control of the federal government, new federal legislation banning abortion faces an uphill battle because of the Senate filibuster. However, if sufficiently motivated, a Republican majority in the Senate could eliminate the filibuster (generally or just for an abortion bill). That would be a stark break from past practice, but it is certainly within the realm of possibility for a party disappointed that *Dobbs* did not more seriously limit abortion in the country.

Even without passing a nationwide abortion ban, a Republican antiabortion president could still have a huge impact on abortion. The next president could very likely have the opportunity to nominate one or more Supreme Court justices. In fact, speculation is growing that if Donald Trump wins in 2024, Justices Clarence Thomas and Samuel Alito, both in their mid-seventies and both conservatives who were part of the *Dobbs* majority, might step aside so they can be replaced with much younger conservative justices who would hold the position for several more decades, further cementing the conservative supermajority on the Court.

An emboldened conservative Court might then move the law closer to finding constitutional "personhood" for fetuses, a longstanding goal of the antiabortion movement. If a future Court does eventually declare fetuses to be constitutional persons, this ruling could mean that all states are required to prohibit abortion in order to provide equal protection to those fetal persons. In other words, a Court declaring fetal personhood could result in a nationwide ban on all abortion, even in states that have put protections for abortion in their own laws or constitutions.

Scarier still, it's possible that a Republican president wouldn't even need a new law or new Supreme Court ruling to seriously curtail or even ban abortion nationwide. An antiabortion president could put like-minded people in charge of the FDA and the Department of Health and Human Services. These administrative officials could cut back accessibility of mifepristone and push American health policy against abortion through agency action, without any need for Congress to act.

Similarly, an antiabortion president could appoint an attorney general who uses the Comstock Act to try to end abortion everywhere in the country. The Comstock Act, a federal law from 1873, bans, among many other things related to sex, mailing any item intended to induce an abortion.[38] The law was passed at a time when women couldn't vote and were considered under law to be the property of their husbands and has not been enforced for almost a century because federal courts have long interpreted it to apply to illegal abortion only. However, since *Dobbs*, the antiabortion movement has been making more and more noise that the Justice Department, if Trump were to win, should enforce the law now, in the twenty-first century, to ban all products that can be used to induce even legal abortions. This interpretation, rejected by the Biden administration, could apply not only to abortion pills but also to instruments and supplies used for procedural abortion. If no abortion provider or clinic could receive these items in the mail or via private express mail services, abortion would be effectively shut down in this country, and Congress wouldn't have to pass any new law to do so.

Of course, a Democratic win in 2024 would mean no nationwide abortion ban, no new conservative Supreme Court justices, and no reinvigoration of the Comstock Act. A Harris administration would at the very least keep the status quo and would not work to disrupt the important gains being made in states that support abortion rights. And if circumstances aligned, a Harris administration could also mean the enactment of statutory protection for abortion nationwide, the end of the Hyde Amendment (which bans Medicaid funding for abortion), and the appointment of new pro-choice justices to the Supreme Court, possibly even replacing some of the Court's antiabortion conservatives. Which of these candidates wins in 2024 will make a significant difference for everyone involved with abortion.

THE ULTIMATE ISSUE: SUSTAINABILITY

Regardless of which party's candidate ends up in the Oval Office, what happens next is unknown. As should be evident from all of the stories throughout this book, the work required to make abortion possible in the wake of *Dobbs*—in even greater numbers than before—is both difficult and costly. That means that a hugely consequential question going forward, the one that will play a huge role in determining whether what we have chronicled in the immediate aftermath of *Dobbs* becomes the new steady-state reality, is the sustainability of everything we cover in this book.

For now, those people who are less directly involved than the providers and advocates in this book but who agree that the overturning of *Roe* was unacceptable have stood up and engaged in the struggle to make abortion as accessible as possible and to ease the burden on patients and providers alike. They have contributed financially to abortion funds, which always have more requests of help than they can meet; they have driven patients who have transportation challenges; they have escorted at clinics to shield patients from aggressive protesters; and they have voted with abortion on their minds, in every election, not just presidential ones, and for every position on the ballot, including in state and local races. People have also spoken out in favor of abortion rights in all sorts of venues, such as op-eds, letters to the editor of local papers, call-ins to radio programs, and wherever else the opportunity presents itself. If the overturning of *Roe* has revealed anything, it is that the American people want abortion to remain available and have taken it upon themselves to speak about how important this healthcare option is and to act to defend it. Anyone who continues to feel this way about the importance of abortion access, rights, and justice needs to continue to act accordingly, even in the face of outrage fatigue and a seemingly long battle ahead.

Because without a continued influx of money,[39] time, and resources to support abortion travel and funding; without providers continuing to be able to work tireless hours and every angle to provide care to everyone who comes to them; without innovators continuing to be willing to push the envelope with abortion pill distribution channels and new service delivery models; and without lawyers, advocates, and elected officials working to block even more states making abortion illegal or severely limited in the future and to ensure that operating an abortion clinic in states where the practice remains legal is economically sustainable[40]—there may soon come a time when the overturning of *Roe* means a severe decline in the number of people able to obtain the abortions they seek.

Until then, what we have seen so far is that the loss of a national constitutional right has been unjustly disruptive to and taxing on so many people's lives. But because of the incredible work of the people in this book, those like them, and those who support them, even though *Roe* has ended, abortion has not.

EPILOGUE

And then the 2024 election happened.

We write this in the days immediately following the election and months after we finished the rest of this book. With Donald Trump winning the presidency for a second time, the political fears we detail in the last chapter of the book take a big step closer to becoming reality. By the time this book is published and you are reading these words, we will have a better sense of whether President Trump will be enforcing the Comstock Act, cutting back on or even eliminating FDA approval for mifepristone, and taking steps to limit abortion-related travel.

By the time this book is published, we will also know who controls Congress. As of now (mid-November 2024), we know that Republicans will have a clear majority in the Senate, but control of the House remains up in the air. If Republicans take control of both houses, the prospect of national legislation banning abortion will materialize. In order for that to happen, the Senate would have to eliminate the filibuster and President Trump would have to go back on his 2024 campaign statements that he would not sign a national ban, but both are entirely possible. However, if the Democrats manage to eke out a majority in the House, we can rest knowing that at least in the next two years there will be no national legislation banning abortion (though the possibility of Comstock enforcement resulting in a de facto national ban would remain).

In state elections, the right to abortion won majorities in eight of the ten states where it was on the ballot. Only in South Dakota and Nebraska did abortion rights fail to reach 50 percent. However, because of Florida's requirements for ballot initiatives, the constitutional amendment also failed there. In that state, a lopsided majority of voters approved the abortion referendum, but it fell three percentage points short of the 60 percent threshold for ballot initiatives. As a result, the right to abortion will be added to the constitution of seven states because of the election: Arizona,

Colorado, Maryland, Missouri, Montana, Nevada, and New York. Arizona and Missouri are the most significant on this list because the amendments expand access in both states—from fifteen weeks to viability in Arizona and from a complete ban to viability in Missouri. In the other states, the election solidifies what was already true on the ground: what was once a right protected by state statute is now a right protected by state constitutional amendment.

These are victories, but they are tempered by the national landscape. If there is a national ban on abortion—via a new federal law or enforcement of the Comstock Act—state constitutional amendments, like state statutes, will fall to the supremacy of federal law. And state constitutional protections would likewise be irrelevant if the FDA cuts back access to mifepristone. Thus, we are back where we started: waiting to see what the new Trump administration does to determine the future of abortion in this country.

Tragically, though, we do know now that, however things play out with national policy as a result of the election, people in states with abortion bans will continue to face forced births, injuries, and even deaths. Shortly after we completed our manuscript, investigative journalists with ProPublica reported on a number of deaths of pregnant women that were directly attributable to the circumstances created by *Dobbs*. The number of these horrific stories will surely grow.

Of course, as with any election, there will be resistance. Though it's looking like Trump won the popular vote, at the end of the day there will possibly be close to seventy-five million people who voted against him. Moreover, given the continued popularity of abortion, in both ballot initiatives and issue polls, a good chunk of the American populace will push back in various ways against any of the efforts we fear may be in the works. We have no idea what the results of this resistance will be, but we do know that the Trump administration's efforts to eviscerate legal abortion will face vigorous opposition.

What we also know is that, despite the results of the 2024 election, the people profiled in this book and others like them are going to do whatever they can to continue to serve the women and other pregnant people who need them. And, even more important, that people who are pregnant in this country and who no longer desire to be so—for whatever reason— will do what they can to get the care they want and need. History has shown this unshakeable determination again and again, as has the story of people throughout the world currently living under abortion bans. Again, we can't know any of the specifics of what this will look like. Will providers switch to misoprostol-only abortions? Will providers and patients rely on foreign distribution of abortion pills? Will patients turn in greater numbers to informal clandestine networks? Will providers of conscience tempt fate and provide abortions that do not comply with new restrictive abortion laws? Only time will tell.

When we researched, wrote, and finalized the main text of this book, we were buoyed by the overarching story of providers, supporters, and patients confronting the new post-*Roe* reality and finding ways to continue on. Our excitement wasn't without caution, as we understood that there was no guarantee that this successful countereffort would last, given political, legal, and financial threats. However, what emerged from this project was, we hope, an inspiring tale of resilience and persistence in the face of injustice.

But the questions we leave you with now, after the 2024 election, are these: Is this book a story of the present *and* the future of abortion under *Dobbs*? Or will this book become a piece of history that captures a unique two-year moment of transition that ends abruptly with the onset of a new political regime? And if this new political regime is as repressive as some fear, can the stories of ingenuity and resistance contained in these pages inform the path forward?

Whatever the answer to these questions, we are confident of this: the deep commitment of the American people to reproductive freedom will certainly mean that the Trump administration's attacks, whatever they are, will not be the last chapter of the abortion story in the United States.

ACKNOWLEDGMENTS

Our greatest debt of course is to the abortion providers—clinicians and clinic administrators alike—and to the advocates and activists who took time out from their extremely busy lives, in an immensely difficult year, to grant our unusual request for three interviews over the course of the year. We hope this book conveys the magnitude of their and their coworkers' achievements, in the face of great odds, in keeping essential healthcare accessible for as many people as possible after the fall of *Roe*.

We are grateful to the following who read all or parts of the manuscript and gave us useful feedback: Greer Donley, Cassie Ehrenberg, Diana Greene Foster, Jill Wieber Lens, Yvette Lindgren, Maya Manian, Rachel Rebouché, Ushma Upadhyay, and Tracy Weitz. We thank our physician friends, Dan Grossman, Maureen Paul, and Shelley Sella, for clarification of some medical issues pertaining to abortion care. We also thank our friends and colleagues at the Abortion Care Network, National Abortion Federation, and Planned Parenthood Federation of America who, although not directly involved in the preparation of this book, have for decades increased our knowledge of both the gratifications and challenges of abortion provision.

At Beacon Press, our editor, Rachael Marks, has been an enthusiastic supporter of this book from the start and a source of excellent advice. At Beacon, we have also enjoyed working with Marcy Barnes, Amy Caldwell, Rebecca Johnson, Frankie Karnedy, Susan Lumenello, Caitlin Meyer, and Mei Su Bailey. It is a pleasure to work with a press whose values around reproductive freedom align with ours. We also thank Kate Scott for copyediting our manuscript.

From David: I am very fortunate to have multiple professional homes that support all the work I do. My full-time job is as a professor at the Drexel Kline School of Law, where everyone has fully been behind everything I do related to abortion, despite the controversies surrounding the topic. Deans Dan Filler, Deborah Gordon, and Amy Landers have provided me not only with leave time and financial support when needed but also encouragement and guidance every step of the way. Thank you as well to the rest of my colleagues who are also always there for assistance, advice, and as a sounding board. My student Lia Knox-Hershey provided excellent research support.

Beyond Drexel, I continue to work on reproductive rights and justice issues in Pennsylvania (and beyond) with the Women's Law Project, where I started my legal career. Susan Frietsche and Carol Tracy have been instrumental in everything I've done that touches on abortion, and the same is true with the work in this book. Everyone at that organization, as well as our clients and others in the Philadelphia-area reproductive rights and justice community, has also contributed to what I know about this topic. And my wonderful coauthors for my more traditional legal scholarship, Greer Donley and Rachel Rebouché, have been essential to helping me figure out everything law-related about (and staying sane in) the post-*Dobbs* landscape.

From Carole: I am tremendously fortunate to work with a group of very smart and productive colleagues at the University of California San Francisco, particularly in the ANSIRH (Advancing New Standards in Reproductive Health) program and the Bixby Center for Global Reproductive Health, both housed in the Department of Obstetrics, Gynecology and Reproductive Sciences. I am particularly grateful to ANSIRH's leadership, Dan Grossman and Molly Battistelli, for providing us with such a rich work environment. And I thank Clare Stewart of ANSIRH for her numerous helpful acts during the writing of this book. David and I both appreciate Paul Garton and his staff at Home Row for their excellent job of transcribing our interviews. I thank my "repro squad," Rivka Gordon, Maureen Paul and Suzan Goodman, for many years of conversations about various aspects of reproductive politics and services.

We both thank our families for their love, support, and valuable feedback throughout this project (and all of our others). Carole thanks Fred, Miriam, Andrew, Jude, Braden, Karl, Jennifer, and Joe. David thanks Cassie, Josh, Leo, Rachel, Seth, Marcia, Arnie, John, and Kathleen. Without all of them, we couldn't do this work.

NOTES

INTRODUCTION

1. On the Ohio story, see J. D. Ruck, "Was the '10-Year-Old Rape Victim Denied Abortion' Story Manufactured?" *America First,* July 6, 2022, https://perma.cc /V496-PTQC; Shari Rudavsky and Rachel Fradette, "Patients Head to Indiana for Abortion Services as Other States Restrict Care," *Indianapolis Star,* July 1, 2022; David Folkenflik and Sarah McCammon, "A Rape, an Abortion, and a One-Source Story: A Child's Ordeal Becomes National News," NPR, July 13, 2022, https:// perma.cc/TC4F-2Y6N; Sarah McCammon and Becky Sullivan, "Indiana Doctor Says She Has Been Harassed for Giving an Abortion to a 10-Year-Old," NPR, July 26, 2022, https://perma.cc/CS69-C22F; Sarah McCammon, "Doctor Told the State She Performed Abortion on 10-Year-Old, Document Shows," NPR, July 15, 2022, https://perma.cc/A5MJ-EXWM; Farah Yousry, "IU Health: Dr. Bernard Complied with Patient Privacy Laws Regarding 10-Year-Old's Abortion," WFYI Indianapolis, July 15, 2022, https://perma.cc/7LZY-5EEA; Marilyn Odendahl, "Medical Licensing Board Hearing on Rokita Complaint Against Bernard Postponed to May 25," *TheStatehouseFile.com* (online magazine), Feb. 13, 2023, https://perma.cc/6X68 -VM3W; Johnny Magdaleno, "'Proud of the Stand I Took': Dr. Caitlin Bernard Will Not Fight Medical Board's Penalty," *Indianapolis Star,* July 29, 2023, https://perma .cc/2JWN-K2F3; "Man Gets Life Sentence for Raping 9-Year-Old Ohio Girl Who Traveled to Indiana for Legal Abortion," Associated Press and Spectrum News 1, July 6, 2023, https://perma.cc/2B3P-YK9H; Bill Chappell, "Indiana High Court Reprimands AG for Remarks About 10-Year-Old Rape Victim's Doctor," NPR, Nov. 3, 2023, https://perma.cc/DXV9-B4D5.

2. 597 U.S. 215 (2022).

3. 597 U.S. 1 (2021).

4. 505 U.S. 833 (1992).

5. Preterm Cleveland v. Yost, No. 19-cv-00360. 2022 U.S. Dist. LEXIS 112700, at *5 (S.D. Ohio June 24, 2022).

6. David S. Cohen and Carole Joffe, *Obstacle Course: The Everyday Struggle to Get an Abortion in America* (Oakland: University of California Press, 2020).

7. Shari Rudavsky and Rachel Fradette, "Patients Head to Indiana for Abortion Services as Other States Restrict Care," *Indianapolis Star,* July 1, 2022, https://perma .cc/4K6D-FGLM.

8. Chappell, "Indiana High Court Reprimands AG for Remarks About 10-Year-Old Rape Victim's Doctor."

9. On Ellie's story and the details about Arizona, see Tiffany Stanley, "After Abortion Protections Fell, Their Lives Were Upended," *Washington Post,* Nov. 30,

2022; Andrew Jeong, "Arizona Court Halts Enforcement of Near-Total Abortion Ban," *Washington Post*, Oct. 8, 2022, https://perma.cc/63DX-PZ8D; Marielle Kirstein et al., "100 Days Post-*Roe*: At Least 66 Clinics Across 15 US States Have Stopped Offering Abortion Care," Guttmacher Institute, Oct. 6, 2022, https://perma.cc /WD5R-FSB9; Tracy Abiaka, "Arizona Providers, Regulators Can't Agree on Abortion Law After *Dobbs*," *Cronkite News*, June 27, 2022, https://perma.cc/9F3K-BHS7; Andrew Oxford, "The Future of Arizona's Abortion Ban Is Back in a Tucson Court," AZPM, Aug. 18, 2022, https://perma.cc/P76X-9NM7.

10. Sarah C. M. Roberts et al., "Risk of Violence from the Man Involved in the Pregnancy After Receiving or Being Denied an Abortion," *BMC Medicine* 12 (Sept. 2014): 144.

11. Isaacson v. Brnovich, 610 F. Supp. 3d 1243, 1257 (D. Ariz. 2022); Planned Parenthood Center of Tucson, Inc. v. Brnovich, No. 127867 (Ariz. Super. Ct. Sept. 22, 2022); Planned Parenthood Arizona, Inc. v. Brnovich, No. C127876 (Ariz. Ct. App. Oct. 7, 2022).

12. On Amanda's story, see *The Assault on Reproductive Rights in a Post-*Dobbs *America, Before the U.S. Senate Committee on the Judiciary*, 118th Cong. (2023) (statement of Amanda Zurawski), https://perma.cc/B6ZS-XQAT; Plaintiff's Original Petition for Declaratory Judgment and Application for Permanent Injunction at 4–8, Zurawski v. State of Texas (Tex. argued Nov. 28, 2023) (No. 23-0629), https:// perma.cc/LZ2J-BCAE; A. J. McDougall, "Texas Woman Who Nearly Died Tears into Ted Cruz at Abortion Hearing," *Daily Beast*, Apr. 26, 2023, https://perma.cc /LSH5-KGAM.

13. Texas v. Zurawski, 690 S.W. 3d 644 (Tex. 2024).

14. National Abortion Federation, "Abortion After *Roe*," https://perma.cc /WM73-WLL3.

15. Jessica Ravitz, "Mississippi Bans Abortions at 15 Weeks, Earliest in the Nation," CNN, Mar. 19, 2018, https://perma.cc/8K42-C3RK.

16. 579 U.S. 582, 627 (2016).

17. Justice Anthony M. Kennedy, letter to President Donald Trump, US Supreme Court, June 27, 2018, https://www.supremecourt.gov/publicinfo/press/letter_to _the_president_june27.pdf.

18. 140 S. Ct. 2103 (2020).

19. Jackson Women's Health Org. v. Currier, 349 F. Supp. 3d 536 (S.D. Miss. 2018).

20. Dobbs v. Jackson Women's Health Organization, 597 U.S. at 348–49 (Roberts, J., concurring).

21. Elizabeth Nash and Isabel Guarnieri, "Six Months Post-*Roe*, 24 US States Have Banned Abortion or Are Likely to Do So: A Roundup," Guttmacher Institute, Jan. 10, 2023, https://perma.cc/7VSG-CJ8K.

22. Nash and Guarnieri, "Six Months Post-*Roe*, 24 US States Have Banned Abortion or Are Likely to Do So."

23. Society of Family Planning, "#WeCount Report," Apr. 11, 2023, https:// perma.cc/4QSB-29S3.

24. Guttmacher Institute, "Monthly Abortion Provision Study," https://perma.cc/5JE3 -W3PC, accessed June 28, 2024; Isaac Maddow-Zimet and Candace Gibson, "Despite Bans, Number of Abortions in the United States Increased in 2023: Monthly Abortion Provision Study," Guttmacher Institute, Mar. 2024, https://perma.cc/8PVY-CSS6.

25. S.B. 8, 87th Leg., 3rd Spec. Sess. (Tex. 2021).

26. Diana Greene Foster, *The Turnaway Study: Ten Years, a Thousand Women, and the Consequences of Having—or Being Denied—an Abortion* (New York: Scribner, 2020).

CHAPTER ONE: OVERTURNING *ROE V. WADE*

1. Dobbs v. Jackson Women's Health Org., 597 U.S. 215 (2022); Roe v. Wade, 410 U.S. 113 (1973).

2. *Roe*, 410 U.S. at 129.

3. U.S. Constitution, amend. 14, sec. 1.

4. *Roe*, 410 U.S. at 153.

5. *Roe*, 410 U.S. at 159–60.

6. 410 U.S. 179 (1973).

7. Johanna Schoen, *Abortion After Roe* (Chapel Hill: University of North Carolina Press, 2015), 23–59.

8. H.B. 1211, 95th Leg., 2nd Reg. Sess. (Mo. 1974); Pennsylvania Abortion Control Act 35 Pa. Stat. Ann. §§ 6601–6608 (1974); Katherine Anne Malfa, "An Analysis of the 1974 Massachusetts Abortion Statute and a Minor's Right to Abortion," *New England Law Review* 10, no. 2 (1975): 438.

9. Fred Barbash, "Ruling on U.S. Abortion Funding Stands," *Washington Post*, Sept. 17, 1980, https://perma.cc/P9M5-DJS3.

10. 95 Cong. Rec. H19700 (1977) (statement of Rep. Hyde).

11. Planned Parenthood of Central Missouri v. Danforth, 428 U.S. 52 (1976); Colautti v. Franklin, 439 U.S. 379 (1979); Bellotti v. Baird, 443 U.S. 622 (1979).

12. Beal v. Doe, 432 U.S. 438 (1977); Maher v. Roe, 432 U.S. 464 (1977); Poelker v. Doe, 432 U.S. 519 (1977); Harris v. McRae, 448 U.S. 297 (1980); Williams v. Zbaraz, 448 U.S. 358 (1980).

13. Brief for the United States as Amicus Curiae in Support of Appellants, Thornburgh v. American College of Obstetricians & Gynecologists, 476 U.S. 747 (1986) (No. 84-495).

14. 492 U.S. 490 (1989).

15. Webster v. Reproductive Health Services, 492 U.S. at 538 (Blackmun, J., dissenting).

16. Colautti v. Franklin, 439 U.S. 379 (1979); Thornburgh v. ACOG, 476 U.S. 747 (1986).

17. Linda Greenhouse, "Abortion Rights Strategy: All or Nothing," *New York Times*, Apr. 24, 1992.

18. Planned Parenthood v. Casey, 505 U.S. 833 (1992) (No. 91-744), Transcript of Oral Argument.

19. Fawn Vrazo Knight-Ridder, "Supreme Court Grilling Leaves Little Confidence," *Albany Times Union*, Apr. 23, 1992.

20. *Casey*, 505 U.S. at 878.

21. *Casey*, 505 U.S. at 877–78.

22. David S. Cohen and Carole Joffe, *Obstacle Course: The Everyday Struggle to Get an Abortion in America* (Oakland: University of California Press, 2020).

23. Rachel K. Jones, Marielle Kirstein, and Jesse Philbin, "Abortion Incidence and Service Availability in the United States, 2020," *Perspectives on Sexual and Reproductive Health* 54, no. 4 (Dec. 2022): 134–35.

24. Rebecca Wind, "Abortion Patients More Likely to Be Poor in 2014 Than in 2008," Guttmacher Institute, May 10, 2016, https://perma.cc/G9XH-LPC2.

25. Whole Woman's Health v. Jackson, 141 S. Ct. 2494, 2495 (2001).

26. *Whole Woman's Health*, 141 S. Ct. at 2498 (Sotomayor, J., dissenting).

27. Whole Woman's Health v. Jackson, 595 U.S. 30 (2021); Whole Woman's Health v. Jackson, 642 S.W. 3d 569 (Tex. 2022).

28. Josh Gerstein and Alexander Ward, "Supreme Court Has Voted to Overturn Abortion Rights, Draft Opinion Shows," *Politico*, May 2, 2022.

29. James D. Robenalt, "The 1973 *Roe v. Wade* Decision Also Was Leaked to the Press," *Washington Post*, May 2, 2022.

30. *Dobbs*, 597 U.S. at 268.

31. *Dobbs*, 597 U.S. at 364 (Breyer, J., Sotomayor, J., and Kagan, J., dissenting).

32. *Dobbs*, 597 U.S. at 372 (Breyer, J., Sotomayor, J., and Kagan, J., dissenting).

33. *Dobbs*, 597 U.S. at 332 (Thomas, J., concurring).

34. *Dobbs*, 597 U.S. at 363 (Breyer, J., Sotomayor, J., and Kagan, J., dissenting).

CHAPTER TWO: CLINIC CLOSURES

1. Marielle Kirstein et al., "100 Days Post-*Roe*: At Least 66 Clinics Across 15 US States Have Stopped Offering Abortion Care," Guttmacher Institute, Oct. 6, 2022, https://perma.cc/T49V-3DZC.

2. Allison McCann and Amy Schoenfeld Walker, "One Year, 61 Clinics: How *Dobbs* Changed the Abortion Landscape," *New York Times*, June 22, 2023.

3. 579 U.S. 582 (2016); 595 U.S. 30 (2021).

4. H.B. 2, 83rd Leg., 2nd Spec. Sess. (Tex. 2013).

5. McCann and Schoenfeld Walker, "One Year, 61 Clinics."

6. Verified Complaint for Declaratory and Injunctive Relief, West Alabama Women's Center et al., v. Marshall et al., No. 2:23-cv-00451 (M.D. Ala. July 31, 2023), https://perma.cc/YQ3G-78EK.

7. David S. Cohen and Carole Joffe, *Obstacle Course: The Everyday Struggle to Get an Abortion in America* (Oakland: University of California Press, 2020), 8; Kristina Tocce and Britt Severson, "Funding for Abortion Training in Ob/Gyn Residency," *AMA Journal of Ethics* 14, no. 2 (Feb. 2012): 113–14.

8. Sarah Horvath et al., "Increase in Obstetrics and Gynecology Resident Self-Assessed Competence in Early Pregnancy Loss Management with Routine Abortion Care Training," *Obstetrics & Gynecology* 139 no. 1 (Jan. 2022): 116–19.

9. UNC Health and UNC School of Medicine, "Researchers Document Health Provider Impacts from Post-*Dobbs* Abortion Bans," Jan. 17, 2024, https://perma.cc/NZ2M-FKWB.

CHAPTER THREE: CREATIVE ALTERNATIVES

1. Jesse Bedayn, "A Woman Pleads Guilty to Fire That Kept a Wyoming Abortion Clinic from Opening for a Year," Associated Press, July 20, 2023, https://apnews.com/article/wyoming-abortion-clinic-fire-bf23a8e3bd37c429a274b4e16cf2607f.

2. H.B. 92, 66th Leg. (Wyo. 2022).

3. Kate Zernike, "Wyoming Banned Abortion. She Opened an Abortion Clinic Anyway," *New York Times*, Mar. 14, 2024; Pam Belluck, "Wyoming Judge Temporarily Blocks the State's New Abortion Ban," *New York Times*, Mar. 22, 2023.

4. Livia Albeck-Ripka, "Arsonist Ordered to Pay Nearly $300,000 for Damages to Wyoming Abortion Clinic," *New York Times*, Dec. 27, 2023.

5. Clair McFarland, "Casper Mayor Gives Emotional Apology for Abortion Hellfire Post, Says He Won't Resign," *Cowboy State Daily*, May 2, 2023, https://perma.cc/L2P4-SRES.

6. Carole E. Joffe, *Doctors of Conscience: The Struggle to Provide Abortion Before and After Roe v. Wade* (Boston: Beacon Press, 1995).

7. Jon Wiener and Eyal Press, "Are the Risk Managers Running Planned Parenthood?" *The Nation*, May 30, 2023, https://www.thenation.com/article/activism/sms-press-qa-planned-parenthood/.

8. Emily Witt, "An Abortion Clinic One Year Later," *New Yorker*, June 23, 2024, https://www.newyorker.com/news/us-journal/an-abortion-clinic-one-year-later.

CHAPTER FOUR: PIVOT MASTERS

1. Epigraph: "Quotation of the Day: Strategic Shift in Bid to Regain Abortion Rights," *New York Times*, July 4, 2022; Adam Serwer, "The Cruelty Is the Point," *The Atlantic*, Oct. 3, 2018.

2. FDA v. All. For Hippocratic Med., 144 S. Ct. 537 (2023); Idaho v. United States, 144 S. Ct. 541 (2024).

3. Claire Cain Miller, Quoctrung Bui, and Margo Sanger-Katz, "Abortions Fell by Half in Month After New Texas Law," *New York Times*, Oct. 29, 2021.

4. Order on Motion for Partial Judgment on the Pleadings and Motion to Dismiss, SisterSong Women of Color Reproductive Justice Collective v. State of Georgia, No. 2022CV357796 (2022), https://perma.cc/6RBU-JYVQ.

5. State of Ga. v. SisterSong Women of Color Reproductive Justice Collective, 317 Ga. 528, 544 (2023); ACLU, "Georgia Supreme Court Allows Six-Week Abortion Ban to Again Take Effect," press release, Nov. 23, 2022, https://perma.cc/RUH6-PV5T.

6. S.B. 174, 63rd Leg. (Utah, 2020).

7. Greer Donley and Caroline M. Kelly, "Abortion Disorientation," *Duke Law Journal* 74 (2024).

8. H.B. 481, 155th Leg. (Ga. 2019).

9. Isaacson v. Brnovich, 610 F. Supp. 3d 1243, 1256 (D. Ariz. 2022).

10. 18 U.S.C. §§ 1461, 1462.

11. David S. Cohen, Greer Donley, and Rachel Rebouché, "Abortion Pills," *Stanford Law Review* 76, no. 2 (Feb. 2024): 354; Saige Miller, "Utah Lawmakers Send 'Cease-and-Desist' Demands to Abortion Providers and Advocates," KUER, Sept. 16, 2022, https://perma.cc/FS4Y-BQ3B.

12. Patricia Mazzei, "Florida's Six-Week Abortion Ban Is Now Law, with Political Implications," *New York Times*, May 1, 2024.

13. S.B. 20, 156th Leg. (N.C. 2023); Kelly Baden, Talia Curhan, and Joerg Dreweke, "In the First Month After North Carolina's Latest Abortion Restrictions, Facility-Based Abortions Dropped by 31%," Guttmacher Institute, Oct. 11, 2023, https://perma.cc/8DRP-FXVN.

14. A Woman's Choice, "We are proud to announce that A Woman's Choice clinics have expanded services to Danville, VA!" announcement, Feb. 22, 2024, https://perma.cc/9X2H-8YKD.

CHAPTER FIVE: SURGE STATES

1. Isaac Maddow-Zimet et al., "New State Abortion Data Indicate Widespread Travel for Care," Guttmacher Institute, Sept. 7, 2023, https://perma.cc/TH4H-BXGH.

2. Maddow-Zimet et al., "New State Abortion Data."

3. Susan Dunlap, "Planned Parenthood Clinics in New Mexico Expand, Offering Medication Abortion Care at All Locations," *New Mexico Political Report*, June 6, 2023, https://perma.cc/3TES-KTMY.

4. FDA v. All. For Hippocratic Med., 144 S. Ct. 537 (2023).

5. Sophie Putka, "Planned Parenthood of New Mexico Limits Non-Abortion Care Due to Surge from Texas," *Med Page Today*, Aug. 18, 2023, https://perma.cc /92BJ-GEQK.

6. Carol Mason, "How Trumpism Fostered Anti-Choice Violence," *Ms.*, Feb. 2, 2021, https://perma.cc/2CGE-NMSM.

7. American College of Obstetricians and Gynecologists, "Medication Abortion Up to 70 Days of Gestation," *ACOG Practice Bulletin*, no. 225 (March 2014), reaffirmed 2023, https://www.acog.org/clinical/clinical-guidance/practice-bulletin /articles/2020/10/medication-abortion-up-to-70-days-of-gestation.

8. David S. Cohen and Carole Joffe, *Obstacle Course: The Everyday Struggle to Get an Abortion in America* (Oakland: University of California Press, 2020), 209–13.

9. University of Illinois College of Medicine, Department of Obstetrics and Gynecology, "Announcing the Coordination Service for Hospital-Based Abortion Care (CARLA) Program," press release, Nov. 19, 2022, https://perma.cc/4CWX-2U8C.

10. Advancing New Standards in Reproductive Health (ANSIRH), "Trends in Abortion Facility Gestational Limits Pre- and Post-*Dobbs*," University of California, San Francisco, June 20, 2023, https://perma.cc/5E5L-663F.

11. David S. Cohen and Krysten Connon, *Living in the Crosshairs: The Untold Stories of Anti-Abortion Terrorism* (Oxford: Oxford University Press, 2015), 207–11.

12. James Risen and Judy L. Thomas, *Wrath of Angels: The American Abortion War* (New York: Basic Books, 1998), 75–76.

13. Elevated Access, "We Believe Everyone Deserves Access to Healthcare," https://perma.cc/4KZW-JWNU, accessed June 28, 2024.

14. Ben Brazil, "Planned Parenthood Medical Director, a Former Fighter Pilot, Began Flying Through Gender Barriers as a Girl," *Daily Pilot*, Aug. 29, 2019, https:// perma.cc/9RDR-2P9T.

15. Janet Jacobson, "Commentary: This Is What the End of *Roe* Looks Like in Southern California," *Daily Pilot*, June 28, 2022, https://perma.cc/H5MQ-49GH.

16. Office of Governor Gavin Newsom, "California Expands Access and Protections for Reproductive Health Care," press release, Sept. 27, 2023, https://perma .cc/8RKC-FSV8.

17. "Complex Family Planning Fellowship," Society of Planning, https://perma .cc/TM4C-33EG, accessed June 28, 2024.

18. Andrew Jeong, "Arizona Court Halts Enforcement of Near-Total Abortion Ban," *Washington Post*, Oct. 8, 2022, https://perma.cc/63DX-PZ8D.

19. Kimya Forouzan, Amy Friedrich-Karnik, and Isaac Maddow-Zimet, "The High Toll of US Abortion Bans: Nearly One in Five Patients Now Traveling Out of State for Abortion Care," Guttmacher Institute, Dec. 7, 2023, https://perma .cc/36ZC-QQN8.

20. Almost a year after our last interview with Mercedes, she became the organization's executive director.

21. David S. Cohen and Carole Joffe, "Anti-Choice Politicians Are Using the Coronavirus Crisis to Deny Abortion Rights," *Rolling Stone*, Mar. 25, 2020, https://www.rollingstone.com/politics/political-commentary/anti-choice-politicians-are-using-the-coronavirus-crisis-to-deny-abortion-rights-973096/.

22. Alison Saldanha, "Abortions Jump 23% in WA as Visiting Patients Reverse Decadelong Decline," *Seattle Times*, Dec. 6, 2023, https://perma.cc/6J2Z-ZNNW.

23. David S. Cohen, Greer Donley, and Rachel Rebouché, "Abortion Shield Laws," *New England Journal of Medicine Evidence* 2, no. 4 (2023).

CHAPTER SIX: PILLS

1. Rachel K. Jones and Amy Friedrich-Karnik, "Medication Abortion Accounted for 63% of All US Abortions in 2023—An Increase from 53% in 2020," Guttmacher Institute, Mar. 19, 2024, https://perma.cc/S34V-3THH.

2. Rachel Roubein, "The Fight over Medication Abortion Is Just Getting Started," *Washington Post*, Nov. 29, 2022, https://perma.cc/L3V6-VYC6.

3. R. D. Glasgow, "Chemical Warfare on the Unborn Takes Many Forms," *National Right to Life News* 15, no. 21 (Nov. 17, 1988): 9.

4. Heidi Moseson et al., "Effectiveness of Self-Managed Medication Abortion Between 9 and 16 Weeks of Gestation," *Obstetrics & Gynecology* 142, no. 2 (Aug. 2023): 334.

5. FDA v. Am. Coll. of Obstetricians & Gynecologists, 141 S. Ct. 578, 578–85 (2021).

6. US Food & Drug Administration, "Information About Mifepristone for Medical Termination of Pregnancy Through Ten Weeks Gestation," current as of March 23, 2023, https://www.fda.gov/drugs/postmarket-drug-safety-information-patients-and-providers/information-about-mifepristone-medical-termination-pregnancy-through-ten-weeks-gestation.

7. Priya Anand, "Abortion Pill Startup Choix Raises $1 Million in Venture Capital," Bloomberg.com, June 3, 2022, https://www.bloomberg.com/news/articles/2022-06-01/abortion-pill-startup-choix-raises-1-million-in-venture-capital.

8. Julia McReynolds-Pérez et al., "Ethics of Care Born in Intersectional Praxis: A Feminist Abortion Accompaniment Model," *Journal of Women in Culture and Society* 49, no. 1 (Autumn 2023).

9. David S. Cohen, Greer Donley, and Rachel Rebouché, "Abortion Pills," *Stanford Law Review* 76, no. 2 (Feb. 2024).

10. Caroline Kitchener, "Blue-State Doctors Launch Abortion Pill Pipeline into States with Bans," *Washington Post*, July 19, 2023, https://perma.cc/KC4W-NW4A; Pam Belluck, "Abortion Shield Laws: A New War Between the States," *New York Times*, Feb. 22, 2024.

11. Amelia Bonow, Facebook, Sept. 19, 2015, 3:10 p.m., https://perma.cc/YE72-9FZU.

12. Maria L. La Ganga, "Why the Founder of #ShoutYourAbortion Had to Go into Hiding," *Los Angeles Times*, Sept. 30, 2015, https://perma.cc/CL8Z-9S42.

13. Caroline Kitchener, "Self-Managed Abortion Could Be the Future—But It's Very Hard to Talk About," *Washington Post*, Dec. 20, 2021.

14. Society of Family Planning, "#WeCount Report," June 15, 2023, https://perma.cc/XT5K-E9RS.

CHAPTER SEVEN: SUPPORTING PATIENTS

1. David S. Cohen and Carole Joffe, *Obstacle Course: The Everyday Struggle to Get an Abortion in America* (Oakland: University of California Press, 2020).

2. Harris v. McRae, 448 U.S. 297 (1980).

3. Rachel K. Jones and Amy Friedrich-Karnik, "Medication Abortion Accounted for 63% of All US Abortions in 2023—An Increase from 53% in 2020," Guttmacher Institute, Mar. 19, 2024, https://perma.cc/S34V-3THH; Selena Simmons-Duffin and Shelly Cheng, "How Many Miles Do You Have to Travel to Get Abortion Care? One Professor Maps It," NPR, June 21, 2023, https://perma.cc/SRQ3-UY69.

4. Allie Kelly, "Abortions Now Cost Over $450, More Than Double the Price Before *Roe* Was Overturned, Per a Reproductive Care Nonprofit Director," *Business Insider*, Feb. 29, 2024, https://perma.cc/9NW3-WFTZ.

5. James W. Loewen, *Sundown Towns: A Hidden Dimension of American Racism* (New York: New Press, 2005).

6. Ivette Gomez, Alina Salganicoff, and Laurie Sobel, "Abortions Later in Pregnancy in a Post-*Dobbs* Era," KFF Women's Health Policy, Feb. 21, 2024, https://perma.cc/YS7Y-8ABR.

7. Lana Wilson and Martha Shane, dir., *After Tiller*, Ro*co Films, 2013.

8. Later Abortion Initiative, "Referrals for Abortion Care After 24 Weeks," Oct. 2023, https://perma.cc/4AHF-9BVS.

9. Since we interviewed her, Odile has left Brigid for other opportunities.

10. Kimya Forouzan, Amy Friedrich-Karnik, and Isaac Maddow-Zimet, "The High Toll of US Abortion Bans: Nearly One in Five Patients Now Traveling Out of State for Abortion Care," Guttmacher Institute, Dec. 7, 2023, https://perma.cc/36ZC-QQN8.

CHAPTER EIGHT: ABORTION'S UNCERTAIN FUTURE

1. Guttmacher Institute, "Number of Abortions in the United States Likely to Be Higher in 2023 Than in 2020," press release, Jan. 17, 2024, https://perma.cc/9GA7-VBLY.

2. World Health Organization, "Abortion," May 17, 2024, https://perma.cc/LW9F-ED7J.

3. Daniel Dench, Mayra Pineda-Torres, and Caitlin Knowles Myers, "The Effects of the *Dobbs* Decision on Fertility," IZA Institute of Labor Economics, Discussion Paper Series, no. 16608 (Nov. 2023): 4, https://perma.cc/Y3XG-35LT.

4. Amanda Jean Stevenson, Leslie Root, and Jane Menken, "The Maternal Mortality Consequences of Losing Abortion Access," *SocArXiv*, June 29, 2022, https://perma.cc/XF9E-E94Z.

5. Kira Eidson, "Addressing the Black Mortality Crisis in the Wake of *Dobbs*," *Georgetown Journal of Gender and the Law* 24, no. 3 (2023): 938, https://perma.cc/RSF8-A4L7.

6. Advancing New Standards in Reproductive Health (ANSIRH), "The Turnaway Study," https://perma.cc/3W7F-3PME, accessed June 28, 2024.

7. Camille Kidd, Shaina Goodman, and Katherine Gallagher Robbins, "Issue Brief: State Abortion Bans Threaten Nearly 7 Million Black Women, Exacerbate the Existing Black Maternal Health Crisis," issue brief, National Partnership of Women and Families, May 2024, https://perma.cc/8QZ6-3UEC.

8. Geoff Mulvihill, "What We Know About the Legal Case of a Texas Woman Denied the Right to an Abortion," Associated Press, Dec. 12, 2023, https://perma .cc/A9YD-ZZS7; Eleanor Klibanoff, "Kate Cox's Case Reveals How Far Texas Intends to Go to Enforce Abortion Laws," *Texas Tribune*, Dec. 13, 2023, https://perma .cc/C6DE-UKT9.

9. In re State, No. 23-0994, 2023 Tex. LEXIS 1214, at *2 (Dec. 11, 2023), https:// perma.cc/PM6E-WB4K.

10. Lisa H. Harris, "Navigating Loss of Abortion Services—a Large Academic Medical Center Prepares for the Overturn of *Roe v. Wade*," *New England Journal of Medicine* 386, no. 22 (June 2022): 2061, https://www.nejm.org/doi/full/10.1056 /NEJMp2206246.

11. Greer Donley and Caroline M. Kelly, "Abortion Disorientation," University of Pittsburgh Legal Studies Research Paper No. 2024-04, forthcoming in *Duke Law Journal* 74 (2025), https://ssrn.com/abstract=4729217.

12. Daniel Grossman et al., *Care Post-Roe: Documenting Cases of Poor-Quality Care Since the Dobbs Decision*, report, Advancing New Standards in Reproductive Health (ANSIRH), May 16, 2023. https://www.ansirh.org/research/research/how-post-roe -laws-are-obstructing-clinical-care.

13. Carter Sherman, "Law Protecting Women Seeking Emergency Abortions Is Target in US Supreme Court Case," *The Guardian*, Jan. 9, 2024, https://www .theguardian.com/us-news/2024/jan/09/emergency-abortion-supreme-court-case -emtala-idaho.

14. Stephania Taladrid, "Did an Abortion Ban Cost a Young Texas Woman Her Life?" *New Yorker*, Jan. 8, 2024, https://www.newyorker.com/magazine/2024/01/15 /abortion-high-risk-pregnancy-yeni-glick.

15. Elizabeth G. Raymond and David A. Grimes, "The Comparative Safety of Legal Induced Abortion and Childbirth in the United States," abstract, *Obstetrics and Gynecology* 119, no. 2 (Feb. 2012): 215–19, https://pubmed.ncbi.nlm.nih.gov /22270271/.

16. Warren M. Hern, "Pregnancy Kills. Abortion Saves Lives," *New York Times*, May 21, 2019.

17. Jocelyn Viterna, "Opinion: The Kate Cox Case Shows the Cruelty of Texas' Abortion Law," CNN, updated Mar. 7, 2024, https://perma.cc/D7EX-6PJU.

18. Carole E. Joffe, *Doctors of Conscience: The Struggle to Provide Abortion Before and After* Roe v. Wade (Boston: Beacon Press, 1995).

19. Mary Ziegler, "Lizelle Herrera's Texas Arrest Is a Warning," NBC News, Apr. 16, 2022, https://perma.cc/EL58-FR9T.

20. Jessica Valenti, "No Indictment for Brittany Watts," *Abortion, Every Day* (Substack), Jan. 11, 2024, https://perma.cc/U8NW-UNUK.

21. Grossman et al., *Care Post-Roe*.

22. Pregnancy Justice, "Pregnancy Justice Report Reveals Massive Scope of the Criminalization of Pregnant People," press release, Sept. 19, 2023, https://www .pregnancyjusticeus.org/press/pregnancy-justice-new-report-reveals-massive-scope -of-pregnancy-criminalization/.

23. Katie Watson et al., "Supporting, Not Reporting—Emergency Department Ethics in a Post-*Roe* Era," abstract, *New England Journal of Medicine* 387, no. 10 (Sept. 2022), https://www.nejm.org/doi/10.1056/NEJMp2209312.

24. Erika L. Sabbath, Samantha M. McKetchnie, and Kavita S. Arora, "US Obstetrician-Gynecologists' Perceived Impacts of Post–*Dobbs v. Jackson* State Abortion Bans," *Journal of the American Medical Association* 7, no. 1 (Jan. 2024): 3–5, https://perma.cc/7993-EF69.

25. Kelcie Moseley-Morris, "Idaho Supreme Court Upholds Abortion Ban, Civil Enforcement Law," *Idaho Capital Sun*, Jan. 5, 2023, https://perma.cc/GEV2-7AA8.

26. Rachel Cohen, "Idaho Dissolves Maternal Mortality Review Committee, as Deaths Remain High," Boise State Public Radio News, July 7, 2023, https://perma.cc/ER4L-3LUL.

27. Sheryl Gay Stolberg, "As Abortion Laws Drive Obstetricians from Red States, Maternity Care Suffers," *New York Times*, Sept. 6, 2023.

28. Julianne McShane, "Pregnant with No Ob-Gyns Around: In Idaho, Maternity Care Became a Casualty of Its Abortion Ban," NBC News, Sept. 30, 2003, https://perma.cc/Z5NY-NBWJ. For more information on ob-gyn deserts, see "Academy Pushes Lawmakers to Deliver Rural MOMS Act," *American Academy of Family Physicians*, Aug. 28, 2019, https://www.aafp.org/news/government-medicine/20190828momsact.html.

29. Katy B. Kozhimannil, Peiyin Hung, and Carrie Henning-Smith, "Association Between Loss of Hospital-Based Obstetric Services and Birth Outcomes in Rural Counties in the United States," *Journal of the American Medical Association* 319, no. 12 (Mar. 2018): 1244–45, https://perma.cc/7Z2F-BLXB.

30. McShane, "Pregnant with No Ob-Gyns Around."

31. Brendan Murphy, "After *Dobbs*, M4s Face Stark Reality When Applying for Residency," American Medical Association, July 31, 2023, https://perma.cc/Y2V2-ZV2N.

32. Erika Edwards, "Abortion Bans Could Drive Away Young Doctors, New Survey Finds," NBC News, May 18, 2023, https://perma.cc/6SZT-EBJZ.

33. Moyle v. United States, No. 23-726 (June 27, 2024).

34. All. for Hippocratic Med. v. United States Food & Drug Admin., No. 23-235 (U.S. 2024).

35. Leah R. Koenig et al., "The Role of Telehealth in Promoting Equitable Abortion Access in the United States: Spatial Analysis," abstract, *Journal of Medical Internet Research* 9 (July 2023): 6, https://perma.cc/43EV-AKG2.

36. World Health Organization, "WHO Recommendations on Self-Care Interventions," technical document, "Overview," Sept. 21, 2022, https://perma.cc/FKV3-PQTA; American College of Obstetrics and Gynecologists, "Medication Abortion up to 70 Days of Gestation," *Practice Bulletin* 225, Oct. 2020, https://perma.cc/WQ49-JXJJ.

37. Maggie Astor, "Democrat Running on Abortion and I.V.F. Access Wins Special Election in Alabama," *New York Times*, Mar. 27, 2024, https://www.nytimes.com/2024/03/27/us/politics/alabama-democrat-special-election-ivf.html.

38. David S. Cohen, Greer Donley, and Rachel Rebouché, "Opinion: It's Too Dangerous to Allow This Antiquated Law to Exist Any Longer," CNN, Jan. 22, 2024, https://perma.cc/WBS9-TBKW.

39. Olivia Goldhill, "Abortion Funds Run Short of Money as Demand Soars and Donations Fall," *STAT*, Jan. 23, 2024, https://perma.cc/S6CZ-U3SE.

40. Jennifer Miller, "For Abortion Providers, a Tough Business Gets Even Tougher," *New York Times*, Aug. 17, 2024, https://www.nytimes.com/2024/08/17/business/abortion-clinic-laws.html.

INDEX